# At War with PTSD

# At War with PTSD

Battling Post Traumatic Stress Disorder
with Virtual Reality

Robert N. McLay, M.D., Ph.D.

The Johns Hopkins University Press | Baltimore

© 2012 The Johns Hopkins University Press
All rights reserved. Published 2012
Printed in the United States of America on acid-free paper
9  8  7  6  5  4  3  2  1

The Johns Hopkins University Press
2715 North Charles Street
Baltimore, Maryland 21218-4363
www.press.jhu.edu

Library of Congress Cataloging-in-Publication Data
McLay, Robert N.
At war with PTSD : battling post traumatic stress disorder with virtual reality /
Robert N. McLay.
    p. ; cm.
    Includes index.
    ISBN-13: 978-1-4214-0557-5 (hdbk. : alk. paper)
    ISBN-10: 1-4214-0557-1 (hdbk. : alk. paper)
    ISBN-13: 978-1-4214-0593-3 (electronic)
    ISBN-10: 1-4214-0593-8 (electronic)
    I. Title.
[DNLM: 1. Stress Disorders, Post-Traumatic—therapy—United States. 2. Iraq
War, 2003 —United States. 3. Military Personnel—psychology—United States.
4. Psychotherapy—methods—United States. 5. User-Computer Interface—
United States. WM 172.5]
    616.85'212—dc23          2011042881

A catalog record for this book is available from the British Library.

*Special discounts are available for bulk purchases of this book. For more information, please
contact Special Sales at 410-516-6936 or specialsales@press.jhu.edu.*

The Johns Hopkins University Press uses environmentally friendly book materials,
including recycled text paper that is composed of at least 30 percent post-consumer
waste, whenever possible.

# Contents

Chapter 10.   Women at War   91

Chapter 11.   Memorial Day in Camp Fallujah   99

Chapter 12.   It Just Might Work   109

Chapter 13.   The State of the Science   125

Chapter 14.   Therapy in Foxholes   139

Chapter 15.   The War at Home   153

Chapter 16.   Virtual Reality Faces the Real Thing   163

Chapter 17.   Different Roads Home   175

Chapter 18.   A Kind of Peace: What We Learned and What We Have
             Left to Accomplish   195

             Acknowledgments   201

             Index   203

# At War with PTSD

# Prologue

THE desert wind was picking up as we drove down the main road between the airport and Baghdad. The drive had otherwise been quiet, with only the rumble of the Humvee's diesel engine vibrating through the floorboards. To my right, a statue of Saddam Hussein stood lonely in an otherwise empty stretch of desert. Sand kicked up by a mixture of the weather and the wheels of the convoy made it difficult to make out the stone face, so we drove by unaware of whether the dictator's eyes focused in our direction.

A boom in the distance sounded like a mortar, but my ears were not good enough to tell whether it was friendly or hostile. Smoke rose from the horizon. The Black Hawk helicopter that had escorted us on our path rushed off noisily, presumably going to investigate. The helicopter's departure left us without air cover as we approached an overpass. The whole situation made me nervous, but then so did just about everything here. As Dr. McCoy of *Star Trek* might say, "I'm a doctor, not a combat Marine."

They say you never hear the sound of the gunshot that kills you, but two seconds later, another shell came in with a boom and howl of death. I did not feel the vehicle take the brunt of the impact, but a long crack appeared in the windshield. The Humvee that had been in front of us seemed to vanish, replaced by a smoking heap of rubble. The sound of gunfire was everywhere, interspersed with the loud radio chatter narrating the chaos around us.

"Fire coming in. Fire coming in. One vehicle down. We are in an ambush."

"Are you requesting backup?"

"We are requesting backup! Open fire!"

"Roger. Take evasive action as friendly fire comes in."

I instinctively ducked as something whizzed by, seemingly inches above my head. The world disappeared momentarily into the quiet blackness of the Humvee's interior. When I looked up, we were surrounded. Two men, their faces wrapped in scarves, were standing not fifteen feet from the side of the road. They stood fixed, almost comically exposed, their only defense a suicidal offense of blazing guns.

Why were we not shooting back? The Humvee barreled on, passing within inches of the gunmen, who did not flinch. The whole world turned green, and the Iraqis seemed to flash back and forth between two positions in front of and behind our vehicle.

They hovered there, an endless loop.

"The software still has a few glitches," said Dr. Jim Spira as I took off the headset and returned from virtual Baghdad to the quiet of his San Diego office.

I shrugged. "I'm sure you can fix the bugs, but I still don't understand how this virtual reality stuff is going to help combat Veterans get over post traumatic stress disorder."

# I

# Why This Book Was Written

SERGEANT Bigman was a Ranger, and he lived up to his title and his name. The man was six-foot-six, solid muscle. He came into my office looking angry and irritated to be there. He limped. I was more than a little scared, and I tried not to focus on the earlier words of my boss, Captain K.

"This is one of the best-trained killers on the planet. Everyone else in his unit was slaughtered, and he was captured and tortured by al-Qaeda for weeks. I don't know how he escaped, and I suspect that the men who would have been there to actually see it are dead. He could snap your neck before anyone could get into your office to save you. If that's not enough to make you careful, remember that he's a certified American hero, and every general on the West Coast is looking at what happens to him. So watch what you say."

I started with hello.

He started with, "You know, I never believed in this PTSD stuff. I always thought it was a sorry excuse to get out of work, but I can't sleep. My CO said I had to come and talk to you, so you have one hour, Sir."

I offered him a chair in my cluttered office, noting that even this exceptional man exhibited the familiar mix of irritability restrained by military discipline. The PTSD of which he spoke was post traumatic stress disorder, an affliction the military was trying to get a grip on in the face of ongoing wars in Iraq and Afghanistan. I was one of the Navy's newest-minted so-called experts in the field. I had recently completed a psychiatry residency and, by virtue of having an extra doctorate in stress research, had been placed in charge of a program that tried to push the edges of what we could do for this disorder.

"Your commanding officer can't actually order you to come here," I said. "There are very specific rules for that. You can only be compelled to seek treatment if you are judged to be a danger to yourself or others, and I've not been informed of anything of the like."

"So I can go if I want to?"

"Yes."

He stayed anyway, at least for the hour, plus one more. I'd been given extra time with him because he was, as Captain K had indicated, a certified hero. You could read that from the medals on his chest: a Silver Star, a Purple Heart, and, recently awarded, the Distinguished Service Cross, a decoration second only to the Congressional Medal of Honor. So far, they hadn't handed out that last celestial honor, no matter the acts of valor. On this man's chest, you could see indications of the most note-worthy actions of any Soldier serving. In his eyes, you could see more. This was a true hero and truly human. This was a strong man in pain.

Sergeant Bigman stands out in my mind because he was emblematic of a generation of Service Members—Soldiers, Sailors, Airmen, and Marines—who ended up in my office. He was not the only tough guy to suffer with post traumatic stress disorder. There were many others, some Special Operation supermen like him, others frail from old wounds reopened by the strains of military service. Most were people like you and me, neither tough nor brittle, who had found themselves with terrible events stuck in their heads that dominated their lives.

The military did what it could for these injured men and women. Some people have the impression that PTSD is an incurable tragedy, a mental scar that generals and admirals choose to ignore because it is a battle that cannot be seen and thus could not be won. I can't testify for the entire system, but I will say that at my medical center that wasn't the case. I saw that we could make a difference. Many people got better, went back to their lives, and were stronger for it. But not all.

I never found out the full details of what haunted Sergeant Bigman from the mountains of Afghanistan, although I asked. Avoidance is the second part of PTSD. You re-experience a trauma and try to avoid it, try not to think about it, but running from yourself only makes the memories stronger. As psychiatrists, we try to break that cycle of avoidance, but sometimes we push too hard. Maybe I pushed him away.

"I can't talk about it, not now, not ever," he said, tears brimming on the edge of his scarred face.

He did tell me about growing up rough and hard. Like many sufferers of PTSD, the war was not the beginning of his trauma. His father had beaten him and his brother when they were children, telling them it would make them strong. It had at least pushed them together. He joined the military as an infantry grunt, his brother as a medic. Both ended up in the Special Forces. They had saved each other many times. The action that resulted in his capture was not his first time in combat, not his first time killing or seeing friends die.

"This was worse," he said. "But I didn't think this would happen to me. I was supposed to be stronger than that."

The sergeant had many things going for him that were supposedly protective against PTSD. He was well trained. He had good support from his brother and from his friends. I particularly liked that he was not only tough but also smart. He had earned a college degree before enlisting, and now he had letters of acceptance from several law schools once his term of service was up.

"Why didn't you go in as an officer if you already had a college degree?" I asked. That had been my own path. The military had brought me in as a Navy lieutenant, the third step up in the officer ranks, straight out of medical school. A college degree usually buys you at least the rank of ensign. I couldn't quite fathom why Bigman would have purposefully passed up that advantage.

He practically growled his answer. "In the Special Operation, officers don't get sh--t for action. I wanted to actually do something."

In retrospect, my question had been a mistake. I had insulted his calling, the way that I sometimes felt civilian doctors disdained our volunteer military. Even within the brotherhood of arms, there are often chasms of understanding and respect. In the same way that I was reading his face and his uniform, he had been testing me. And on my own meagerly decorated uniform, the only award was not for serving in combat but rather for publishing academic research. To a man who valued action, I had made myself an outsider.

To Sergeant Bigman everyone had become an outsider. His brother, his fellow Rangers, his country all still loved him. We all wanted to treat him like a hero. But to him, the only people whose respect he wanted, the only people who truly knew his pain, were dead. Some of them, the enemy who had bested him for a time, were slain by his hands. He was struggling not only with PTSD but also with grief, with depression, and with trying to carry the weight of heroism when he felt empty inside.

He had not rejected help altogether. Bigman had avoided alcohol or acting on his anger, traps into which many in his position have fallen. He had befriended a Vietnam Veteran who explained that PTSD was nothing about which to be ashamed. Sergeant Bigman didn't quite believe this, but he did listen. He had even gone so far as to seek out a psychologist whom he had met in survival training school. The psychologist didn't specialize in PTSD, but he was competent and caring. He taught Bigman relaxation techniques and worked with him closely for several months. When the nightmares and flashbacks stubbornly refused to fade, the psychologist suggested to the company commander that perhaps Sergeant Bigman could be given dispensation to travel to Naval Medical Center San Diego, where scientists and physicians were trying out new technologies to help this ancient affliction of war.

Having lost any credibility as a fellow in arms, I tried my best to play up my geek skills. I explained the history of PTSD to Sergeant Bigman, what we had learned about its origins and treatment over the years. I told him what we knew about the underlying biology, but that biology alone was not enough to mend a broken soul. I described how healing the psychological wounds of war involves medicine, psychology, and the fabric of society around us.

"In many ways, PTSD is a normal reaction," I said. "But normal doesn't always mean healthy. It is normal to bleed if you are shot, but that doesn't mean that we should wait forever for a clot to form if you are gushing from the femoral artery. You need medical treatment."

I explained that at this facility in particular we were advancing new work involving virtual reality and other treatments that were making a difference. We had learned what tended to work and what approaches were best avoided. I told him that, even though his story was sure to be unique, I had seen many cases of PTSD. There was nothing here that could not be overcome. I was very optimistic.

I never saw him again.

I started this book thinking that I was writing it for Sergeant Bigman or at least for the others like him, the ones who got away or never came in the first place. I wanted to describe how people with PTSD and other psychological wounds of war can be healed. If people knew this, it seemed like it would help. I wanted a second shot at it. Maybe he, and those like him, would read this. Maybe they would come back.

Later, I realized that writing was also a form of therapy for me. I was waiting to go to Iraq. If someone like Bigman could be broken by war, what chance did I have of returning mentally unscathed? The book took on new meaning, and new chapters formed as I journeyed toward deployment.

On another level, I thought I was writing for other doctors. Psychologists and psychiatrists were interested in the discussions. I wanted to write these thoughts down and to educate the next generation of caregivers. I wanted to make sure that we didn't overlook our past. But there are plenty of books for doctors, enough ways to remember. It is harder to forget.

Sergeant Bigman taught me many things. That isn't his real name, of course, and his story, like all those in this book, has been jumbled and disguised in the writing to protect patient privacy. But it was never really only about him, and it was never just about me.

This book is a collection of what I call psychiatric fables, stories that have a message. My own experiences with science and technology are interspersed with the wisdom and experience of others who have been on the front lines of war and treatment. We will travel back and forth between the battlefield, the ivory tower, and the home front. There are stories from patients, doctors, Service Members, chaplains, family members, neuroscientists, and others. As I gathered information, I appreciated how much I was learning from the process. In the end, I realized that these stories were not about patients or doctors or even friends and family members. They are about war and about healing and about hope. They are about all of us.

# 2

# What Is PTSD Anyway?

## Looking at the Problem before Iraq

IN August of 2001, I was a psychiatry intern at Naval Medical Center San Diego. Not everything you see on TV about being an intern at a big hospital is true, but there is no doubt of two things. You are always exhausted, and you are learning faster than you ever thought possible. We had forty beds on the ward at the time. Each psychiatry resident typically managed between six and twelve patients, all kinds of people: active duty, family members, retired military, the occasional homeless person who had sneaked past the gate. Some were psychotic, some suicidal, some homicidal, others just at the end of their rope. All were asking for our help.

To start this process, we gave them each a diagnosis: *major depressive disorder*, *schizophrenia*, or *bipolar disorder*. As young doctors we lacked personal experience, yet if one individual's depression matched the textbook description, it was not a huge stretch to think treatments the textbook recommended might also be helpful. Each person with a diagnosis also taught us about that condition. It was no exaggeration that our patients were our best instructors. That day in August, my teachers were two patients named John and Maria.

John was a tall, gaunt man, nearing sixty, pale as a ghost and walking like one. His blue eyes looked like they had seen the whole world and

were tired of it. Maria, by contrast, intended to hold the planet responsible. She had the rage of youth, and her heavily accented curses seemed
to fill every moment of time not occupied by sobbing. She was nineteen,
solidly built, and her eyes, though as pained as John's, were dark, danc-
ing, and violent.

Those fiery eyes sparked at a new outrage when Maria and John sat
across from each other in the communal space of Naval Medical Center's
psychiatric ward. They were meeting for morning group.

"How can he have the same f—ing diagnosis as me?" Maria spat.
"These doctors label something, and now you think that is you!"

It was John's introduction that earned Maria's anger. Whereas the
other patients in the circle had shared something of their life story—
Maria had told of her sexual assault, her suicide attempts, and only then
of her diagnoses—John had simply said, "I'm John. I have PTSD."

His response to Maria's challenge was similarly laconic, but the brev-
ity of words came with a torrent of nonverbal expression. He stood to
his full height, the posture a threat. The staff members at the periphery
watched the pair nervously, expecting at any moment to have to break
up a fight. John spoke low, through gritted teeth, "Trust me, darlin', I
ain't sayin' I'm anything like you."

Ironically, in that moment, the mirrored anger made them seem more
alike. I struggled for a way to defuse the situation, stuttered something
about us all getting along. The other patients, more familiar with the
pair, stepped in with humor and insight.

"Hey, you're both in here with us on the psych ward," a young woman
offered, still slightly manic and thus not prone to holding back.

"As I recall, you both drink like fish," another veteran of the ward
offered.

"And neither of you sleeps at night," griped a recent addition to the
psychiatric facility. "You could occasionally remember that other people
do."

The comments invoked another stream of curses from Maria, but her
anger was more diffused now and thus one-on-one combat was avoided.

John sat back down and growled under his breath, "I don't see what
she has to gripe about. I was the one in the damn war."

The war about which John spoke was Vietnam. Afghanistan was not
yet imaginable, and Iraq was still just a place where the Gulf War had

ended quickly and victoriously, leaving relatively few American psychiatric casualties. At that time, John, the Vietnam Veteran, and Maria, the rape victim, represented two archetypes associated with post traumatic stress disorder. They seemed so different, and yet, supposedly, they had much in common. What was it in the origin of their problems, their symptoms, or their responses to treatment that bound these two strangers together under the same diagnosis?

I went back to my office on the ward and opened up a copy of the *Diagnostic and Statistical Manual of Mental Disorders*, or DSM. The DSM has been described as "The Bible" for psychiatrists, but it is nothing so dogmatic. In its simplest form, it is merely lists of symptoms gathered under certain titles, allowing a doctor to determine who does and does not meet the criteria for a diagnosis. For example, according to DSM, a person with major depressive disorder must have a consistently depressed mood for at least two weeks and at least four other symptoms out of eight possibilities. The "statistical" part of the title comes from the way these diagnoses are tested. If a large percentage of these patients can be similarly identified by different doctors in different parts of the country, then a diagnosis is said to be "reliable." If a reasonable number of people so diagnosed seem to have similar natural histories and responses to treatments, then the diagnosis is said to be "valid." Statistically reliable and valid diagnoses remain in the DSM, while others are removed or revised.

PTSD as a diagnosis has had its share of controversy in the DSM. When the manual was first formulated after World War II, much of its development was taken from the *Veterans Administration's Diagnostic Manual*. It was thus natural that *gross stress reaction*, as it was then called, made its way in as a diagnosis in DSM I. When it came time for the manual to be revised to DSM II, however, peace reigned, and this age-old problem was not seen often enough to be considered a reliable diagnosis. By the time DSM III was published, the United States had entered Vietnam. Doctors had again become interested in what afflicted returning warriors. Research criteria for "Vietnam Syndrome" were transformed into the newly titled post traumatic stress disorder.

In flipping through the most recent versions of the tome, I saw that the authors and I wavered on the same issue. Did different forms of trauma really lead to the same condition? Vietnam Syndrome implied something uniquely associated with war. Earlier observers had clearly believed this also. "Shell shock" was thought to be caused by the concussive effects of a large explosion. By the time DSM III had named the condition post traumatic stress disorder, it was clear that the syndrome did not require a blast injury. DSM III listed seventeen possible symptoms that suggested PTSD and required as their cause only a "recognizable stressor that would evoke significant symptoms of distress in almost anyone." DSM-III-R (revised) was more restrictive. It stated that the event must not only be stressful but must also be "outside the range of normal experience." The two most recent versions of the book, DSM IV and DSM IV-TR (text revision), settled on the following requirements:

> The person experienced, witnessed, or was confronted with an event or events that involved actual or threatened death or serious injury, or a threat to the physical integrity of self or others.

> The person's response involved intense fear, helplessness or horror.

I thought about these definitions, and how they might apply to John and Maria. For John, the first part was easy to see. He had been shot at, blown up, stabbed, threatened with torture, and witnessed the deaths of many. He had been, as he put it, "in the damn war." That clearly matched "events that involved actual or threatened death." But what about Maria? She had been raped. Was it the same as a fear of death? Having worked with other rape victims, there was no question that her attack would have involved as much—or more—"fear, helplessness, and horror."

Fear appeared to be a uniting factor. I knew from my days as a basic scientist that the biochemistry of terror had unusual effects on the brain. When an organism is facing death, it throws every resource it has at the situation. In this "fight or flight" response, huge quantities of stress hormones cascade into the body. These can drive muscles to superhuman feats and focus the mind to shut out everything else in the world. But this comes at a price. The same adrenaline that focuses the mind is also linked to anxiety. The cortisol that directs blood sugar to muscles also directs that fuel away from the normal defense of neurons in the memory centers of the brain. Was PTSD just a form of fear burnout?

"I wasn't even scared though," John said when I presented this uni-fying theory to him. "Heck, when I was in 'Nam I was doing fine. It wasn't until I was back in California that things started scaring the sh—t out of me. I know it's totally backwards, but I never flinched at gunfire. Now I hear a loud noise that *sounds* like gunfire and I'm diving for cover."

I pondered this and went back to the books. I also wondered if it were possible not to be scared in combat. I mean, maybe he wasn't aware of how scared he was. The unconscious has fallen out of vogue since the days when psychoanalysis rather than neuroanatomy dominated the reading list of a psychiatry resident. Even those most dismissive of Sigmund Freud and his ideas, however, wouldn't argue that there are thoughts buried deeper than our awareness.

I looked again at the definition of PTSD. The DSM required that to make an accurate diagnosis the patient must have experienced three clusters of symptoms: re-experiencing, avoidance, and an exaggerated state of arousal.

The DSM listed various examples of symptoms that could fall into each of these categories. These were familiar. Maria complained about thoughts and memories never leaving her head. John had nightmares and flashbacks, moments in which, for a second or two, he really thought he was back in Vietnam. Both said that even when they were not thinking about these events, the wrong picture or a smell could send them into fits of fear and make their heart pound in their chests like a bomb.

These symptoms fall into the "re-experiencing" category. This had never made sense to me until I started thinking about what goes on beyond our awareness. Consciously, Maria was thinking about her rape. John's re-experiencing was more subtle. He was haunted in dreams, in visions. Freud and Jung may never have spoken of them, but the most unconscious part of our brain is the oldest, the reptilian core that con-trols pulse and breathing. They might report it in different ways, might even be aware of it on different planes, but both Maria and John had the worst event of their lives burned into their brains. They didn't just remember. It haunted them.

"It wasn't anything you could laugh about," John said, when asked about the events in Vietnam that still came back to him. "Heck, I've

been scared out of my wits plenty of times. All my life, my brother
teased me 'cuz I was afraid of roller coasters, but I don't dream about
roller coasters. I dream about dead kids with their eyes gouged out."

"Yeah, it's the horrible stuff that stays with you," Maria added, finally
softening toward her rival on the ward. "For me, the rape was the most
terrifying moment of my life. But it's more than that. I remember how
scared I was, but what stays with me is not the fear, but the memories
that make me sick and guilty and blame myself. It's like whatever I most
want not to think about, that's the very thing that is in my head twenty-
four seven. I had an abortion after the rape. I couldn't stand the idea
that that bastard's face might show up in my son, follow me around my
whole life. Wouldn't you know it, now I still see his face in every kid I
see. And my damn mother keeps bugging me to have grandchildren. It
doesn't go away."

I nodded. John and Maria were not the only people in the world to
have gone through traumas. But for them, it was that the most unbearable
parts were still there. As DSM would have it, it was not the experiencing
but rather the re-experiencing that made a bad event into PTSD.

With my faith in DSM somewhat bolstered, I pushed ahead to see
if these two also shared commonalities for the second DSM symptom
cluster for PTSD. I asked about avoidance.

Maria was clear on this and explained it with her characteristic flash
of anger. "Of course I avoid things. I told you that I see his face in
every kid. Would you want to get pregnant? Would you want to have
sex again knowing that the man could hurt you? I won't go anywhere
near the place where it happened. I can't even sit in the back seat of a car
anymore. I don't want to think about it. I don't want to talk about it. But
I have to. That's what you damn doctors make me do."

I apologized, a little flustered. Later, I would study more about why
avoidance was so crucial to the perpetuation of PTSD symptoms and how
confronting the trauma and talking about the trauma could take away
its power. This idea formed the basis of the exposure therapy method we
would eventually apply using virtual reality. At the time, however, I was
primarily versed in biological treatments and what we call "supportive
therapy." Supportive therapy involves trying to find ways to make the
patient feel better here and now. Forcing a patient to talk about a trauma

hardly sounded supportive. It seemed to me that avoidance should be classified as a coping technique rather than as a symptom of PTSD.

John jumped in to disabuse me of this idea. It was the longest string of words I had yet to hear come out of his mouth.

"You might have noticed I'm not all that fond of chewin' the fat myself. The one thing I will say for you shrinks though is that talking at the Veterans group did help. I know I cut myself off from things, feelings mostly. I couldn't have emotions, even for my family, because that would mean I had to feel, period. I might not have avoided military bases, but it wasn't a coincidence that my trips there always led to the liquor store. I had to be numb to face the place. Really, I didn't face up to most of my life at all. I didn't think about my future anymore. I even blocked out some of the names of my buddies from Vietnam, and that's what I had promised myself I would never forget."

"So avoidance didn't help you escape the bad memories from the war?" I asked.

"Naw, it's like Maria said. The more you want to get away from something, the more that thing is going to be what you can't get out of your head. It's like you are on a hamster wheel. The faster you run, the faster it turns."

Maria nodded, grudgingly allowing that this might be true. "I guess you can't run away from what's in your own head. You are carrying it around with you."

"Unless you cut it off," John rejoined, the old hostility resurfacing. "That might be about the only place you ain't sliced on yourself darlin'."

Another string of curses flowed between the two.

They certainly had done a good job of displaying the third cluster of PTSD symptoms, the elevated state of irritability and arousal. Anger, anxiety, a tendency to jump out of your chair or off the handle, these were all classified as "persistent symptoms of arousal" by DSM. Also listed, and easily recognized in Maria and John, were insomnia, impaired concentration, and hypervigilance, a tendency always to be on your guard. Judging by the way John had lashed out at Maria, I guessed he had decided it wasn't yet time to let that guard down.

While hospital staff tried once again to calm down the warring pair, I thought about the substance of John's comment. Maria and John had

clearly both shown the three symptom clusters of PTSD: re-experiencing, avoidance, and elevated arousal. Still, DSM mentioned nothing
about suicidal thinking in its definition of PTSD, the very problem that
had landed both John and Maria in the hospital. Nor did DSM include
alcohol or drug abuse in the criteria for post traumatic stress. As other
patients on the ward had pointed out, these were two of the most obvious traits the pair shared. For that matter, they were also problems I had
observed in most PTSD patients who had been on the ward.

It occurred to me that drug abuse and suicidality didn't have to happen. Maybe the reason that Maria and John were both hospitalized, as
opposed to being treated in an outpatient program, was that they were
dealing with additional problems. They had picked up these dangerous
habits as a result, but not as a part, of PTSD. The medical term for this is
*comorbidity.* Comorbidities ride along on PTSD like lampreys on a shark,
but they aren't really part of the same fish.

The hospital staff pulled John and Maria apart. I wished it were as
easy to peel off the comorbidities, the personal conflicts, to see what
was at the heart of the disorder. How many of the problems that PTSD
patients suffered were actually the consequence of PTSD? I could see
how always running from the demons in your head could make it hard
to sleep or to concentrate, but it was difficult to imagine Maria as ever
having been anything but angry.

"Do you think that the anger is from the PTSD?" I decided to ask her
directly, when the situation had calmed. "Or was the fury there first?"

"Part of my personality?" she asked.

"If you want to call it that."

"I don't know. One of the doctors I had before said I had something
called borderline personality disorder, that I had been this way since I
was a kid. They said that I was more angry at my parents for beating me
than I was for the rape that happened later. Psychiatrists seem to think
everything is about your mother, don't they?"

"Do you think it goes back to that?"

"Yeah, well I did have sh–t happen to me as a kid. I admit I was pissed
about it, but I had started to get better. I had hope. Then, when I was
raped, it was like every bad thing I had ever thought about the world was
suddenly proven right."

The picture of Maria's life, in many ways, had been painted long before the sexual assault. Borderline personality disorder is a character type marked by turbulent emotions, bad relationships, and a poor sense of self-preservation, aspects that can mimic PTSD. She might have started off with some of these issues, but even bad lives can get worse. For Maria, the rape had splatter-painted pain across this already messy canvas. Thus, when she saw red, it was hard to tell from which part of the tableau it sprang. But that did not mean that the vandalism had not happened to her soul.

That her personality already included aspects of avoidance and anger only served to isolate her further. She tended to push away people who were trying to help her, and thus, no help was rendered. Her trauma was more personal, an event for which an already poor self-worth made her blame herself. Rape, regardless of the gender or personality of the victim, is the single event most likely to lead to PTSD. Unlike John, who held his trauma in common with thousands of comrades in arms, Maria had no esprit de corps. For her, there was only a dysfunctional family and pain to fall back on.

"That's why I get so mad at John," Maria explained. "I know that we both had bad events change our life. Only, he had a life to begin with."

Ah, envy. But was it accurate? John obviously had better support now. The men from his unit still all stayed in touch, and it sounded like the Veterans group had been good for him. But had it always been this way? Had John, like Maria, found that his traumatic experience awoke demons that were already there?

"Now, I see what you're drivin' at though," John answered when I asked him about this later. "I thought I could guess who was going to come back messed up, too. I never figured it would be me. I was a wild kid, but my folks always taught me I could deal with anything."

"So you had a happy childhood?"

"Real happy. I don't blame my life on anything that happened before the war."

Blame, I thought. Was that what it was all about? Didn't John have to take responsibility for his own life?

John, seeming to detect this thought, answered preemptively. "Now, I'm not sayin' I didn't do anything *after* the war that made things worse."

I nodded. "You're part of AA, which means you acknowledge the consequence of your drinking."

"Yeah, I know about responsibility. One advantage to being in a mental hospital, you do get to see folks who are a lot worse off than you."

"How so?"

"Hey, some of the guys in here, they hear voices. They ramble on like they're on drugs, even when they're not. They have no idea what they're doin'. Not to put too fine a point on it, they're crazy."

"No one says anyone in here is crazy, John." Psychiatrists are not fond of that word. In addition to its pejorative connotation, it doesn't have much scientific validity.

"OK, *insane* then. Some people in here are what you would call insane. I'm not, and neither is Maria."

I acknowledged this. Insane is a legal term used to define someone whose mental illness is so impairing that he or she doesn't know the difference between right and wrong. Most people with a mental illness, including the PTSD sufferers, would not lose touch with reality in this way.

"That makes sense. PTSD is a normal reaction to abnormal events. It doesn't change who you are."

"Oh, that's where you're wrong, Doc. It certainly changes who you are. It makes it easier to fly off the handle and damn harder not to pick up a drink. It's just that you still have some choice in the matter. I don't wake up and decide to feel like life isn't much worth living—that's not the boy my mama raised—but I still get to pick how it all turns out."

I thought about the statistics they had taught us as part of our military psychiatry training to help free us of the myths of Vietnam. Although most vets probably carried bad memories of the war, most were successful in their personal and professional lives. Vietnam Veterans have lower unemployment rates, higher salaries, lower rates of criminal activity, and even lower suicide rates than men and women of the same age who did not go to war. Some of the worst cases of trauma produced the most inspirational stories of recovery.

A few years later everyone would know John McCain, a POW camp survivor, and John Kerry, a three-time Purple Heart recipient, as serious contenders for the presidency. Less well known is the amazing success of many of their comrades. Of the forty-seven men who shared "Room 7" with John McCain in the Hanoi–Hilton torture camp, forty went on to have distinguished military careers after the war. Six of them made admiral or general. That group of survivors now includes congressmen, senators, CEOs, university presidents, a dozen famous authors, and the first man to fly twice the speed of sound. Two Room 7 Veterans received the Medal of Honor. Many went on to lead happy family lives, including one whose daughter grew up to be an astronaut.

Nor was recovery and resilience unique to those who suffered together and wore the American uniform. At least three holocaust survivors have won Nobel Prizes. Celebrities such as Oprah Winfrey and Patty Duke have spoken publicly of abuse they suffered as children. It is generally accepted that the beatings Beethoven received as a boy were linked both to his later deafness and to his famously violent temper.

This is not to say that any of these individuals necessarily suffered from full-blown PTSD. Public speculations have been made about Beethoven and McCain, but there are no hard facts. What is clear is that many people survive trauma, and that, as John had explained, even those with the condition are not doomed to a life in hospitals and clinics. Choices are made, often with great difficulty, but many succeed.

"You seem to have very good insight, John," I said. "And obviously, given your history of service, you have strong discipline and willpower. So if you know what options are better, why do you think that you made so many decisions that caused you pain?"

John indicated empty wrappers on my desk, left over from a rushed "Twinkie lunch." He smiled. "No matter how much you know, sometimes you are bound to take the unhealthy path."

"It's easy to resist anything but temptation," I offered.

"And those temptations are more dangerous when you are already sick. Plenty of my buddies sit around and talk about the war over a beer. For me, the first one feels pretty damn good, but a few hours later, I'm three sheets to the wind and too depressed for anyone to talk to. So do I cut myself off from my friends, or do I end up drunk and locked in a darkened room with my service revolver? Either way, I'm alone and feeling like hell."

"Complicated choices."

He nodded. "PTSD is a complicated thing."

And it is. As John and Maria had shown me, different types of trauma can cause it. Although biology is clearly involved, no lab test or X-ray can diagnose it. We define the problem by the symptoms we see. PTSD has some universal symptoms but can manifest in different ways. How things turn out depends a lot on who you were to begin with, the other problems you pick up along the way, the support you have, and the choices you make. It doesn't render you insane or incapable of doing great things. But it does make everything harder. Every past injury becomes more painful, and every future choice more fraught with peril. Sometimes there will only be the option of the lesser of two evils. It can seem like there is no way out.

"You have to go on living anyway, though," John said.

John and Maria both left the hospital on the same day. John was picked up by a member of the Veterans group that had helped him in the past. Maria, more surprisingly, was driven home by her boyfriend. Despite all her fears about men, she didn't hate them. She wanted a normal life like anyone else and was working hard to get it. This was a tough choice to make but, I'd venture, a good one.

I'd like to say that the pair walked out of the hospital cured. They did not. John was back on the ward a month later. Maria stayed out of the hospital but broke up with her boyfriend and cried about it for hours in therapy. But they lived. Like the old saw goes, where there is life, there is hope. Some things improved, and we learned new ways to help them as time went on. A few of those ways were based on technology and lab research: new medications, new therapies like virtual reality. Most advances occurred the same way that John and Maria moved forward, trial and error. Each step, each mistake or advance, each patient who did well or poorly, each human contact made, they all taught us more.

Three years and a lot of hard work later, Maria married. She still has a temper and fights often with her husband, but she also has a good job, a house in Orange County next to the beach, and a son. She named her firstborn John.

# 3

# Every War Is Different, Every War Is the Same

IRAQ is bordered by Syria, Jordan, Saudi Arabia, Kuwait, Turkey, and Iran. It contains Shiites, Sunnis, Christians, Kurds, Arabs, Assyrians, Iraqi Turkmen, Persians, and others who have managed to simultaneously hate one another and forge great cultures together. Although mostly desert, its central core contains fertile and marshy territory between two of the world's great rivers, the Tigris and the Euphrates. The metropolis of Baghdad is the second-largest city in the Middle East, but vast swaths of the country are inhabited by little but scorpions and desert birds. It is the birthplace of writing and the location of the oldest-known civilization in the world. Iraq is rich in oil but was crushed by poverty, corruption, and the legacy of almost thirty years of warfare. Empires as old as the Babylonians and as recent as the British have tried and failed to hold onto power in Iraq. Iraq was, and was not, what I expected it to be.

I arrived in Camp Fallujah, at the center of Al Anbar province, in February 2008. Our medical team of eight officers and twenty-three enlisted staff climbed out of the convoy trucks to the sounds of clapping and paper horns. It was around three in the morning, but the hospital staff we were replacing had turned out en masse. The doctors, nurses, and corpsmen of Alpha Surgical Company were vigorously celebrating our arrival, and their impending departure, by employing a collection of noisemakers left over from New Year's Eve. As I peered from the back of the seven-ton truck, I was surprised to see something that had almost vanished from memory during the dusty trip across the desert.

"They have trees here," I said, still dazed by the combination of fumes, sleep deprivation, and raucous stimuli. "A lot of trees."

"Well it's not exactly the Pacific Northwest, but, yeah, it doesn't look much like the areas I was in during the Gulf War," agreed Lieutenant Commander Moser, as he helped me maneuver down the back ladder of the truck. "I thought this whole area of the world was one giant stretch of sand."

Norm Moser was a physician assistant assigned to our medical unit, but he had also been our principal guide on military matters as we navigated our way across Kuwait and Iraq. Doc Moser, as he was generally called, was the second-longest-serving member of our team. Both he and our commanding officer joined the Navy at the end of the Vietnam conflict. Unlike the captain, however, Norm had not spent his entire career on the medical side of the military. He had originally served on a destroyer that went upriver in the Mekong Delta and then later become a member of the Navy's elite Special Operations SEAL team before deciding to go back to college to become a physician assistant. You would be hard-pressed to find many individuals with such broad experience.

"So how is this different from the other wars you have been in?" I asked Commander Moser much later when we had settled into our life in Iraq.

"It's a whole different world," he said. "In Vietnam we were demoralized. The mission, the leadership, the traditions, the politics, the public opinions were different, and there were drugs everywhere. In the Gulf War, we were moving so fast that it was over quite quickly once we finally launched the offensive. The whole thing was over before they knew it. Now our troops are better trained, better equipped, and we are all supported."

The support was clearly important. In our own deployment, we had been touched by the generosity of people and organizations back home. It had started even before we left the country. At an airport in Maine, a group of VFW volunteers had braved subzero temperatures in the middle of the night to wish us well on our flight. They did it for every troop-carrying plane that headed to the Middle East. Once in Iraq, friends from whom I had not heard in years sent me packages and e-mail. The packages didn't always do so well on the trip. I started joking that anything sent needed to be treated with the Thanksgiving turkey protocol: place in an oven and bake at 350 degrees for three hours before packaging. Even when a box arrived filled with nothing but a brown stain from melted chocolate that leaked out in the desert, the gift brought a laugh, a sense of connection from home. The very idea that one could send and receive e-mail or text messages in the middle of a war was amazing.

Communication could be, however, a curse as well as a blessing. A sergeant major expounded on the subject when he brought one particularly distraught Marine into the clinic.

"His wife sent him an e-mail." The senior Marine explained about the young man sobbing in the hallway. "We've always had Dear John letters, but now the bad news travels that much faster. Worse, we can't get them away from it. It used to be that when we went into the field for battle, the battle was all you had to worry about. Now, half my Marines are distracted, trying to keep up their relationships, mortgages, and tucking the kids in at night when they should be focused on keeping their heads down."

"But don't you think it is good for morale overall?" I asked when I had finished the session with the heartbroken young man. "The modern communications, I mean."

"Maybe. But when things go wrong, they can go very, very wrong. I've seen awful stuff put up on the Internet. Spouses post videos, messages that are cruel in a way that it is hard to fathom. And it can hurt in both directions. I'm sure you heard on the news about that incident where the soldier's cell phone called his family during the middle of a firefight in Afghanistan."

I had heard about the incident. I also reflected that most of the suicides in theater were related to marital rather than military issues. Freud once famously said that there were two things in life that were truly important to happiness: work and love. Modern warfare means you have to deal with both at once.

There was a lot to deal with in Iraq that had nothing to do with combat but much to do with military life. Even without other people shooting at you, Iraq was dangerous. Eighteen-year-olds were handling explosives and firearms. Military vehicles could flip. Scorpions stung people. The food and water were sometimes contaminated. Strange diseases abounded, and, in 140-degree summer temperatures, people could die from the heat.

For many young men and women convinced of their invulnerability, it wasn't even the danger that was stressful. It was that life was so much out of their control. Orders change on a whim, and suddenly a month-long trip to Kuwait turns into sixteen months in Afghanistan. If you were unfortunate or disliked, the luck could be downright vicious. The military could take your pay and make you keep on working. You could give the system your all, and sometimes the system would still betray you.

After the Vietnam War, the idea arose that isolation and a sense of betrayal caused PTSD. In his book *Achilles in Vietnam*, Jonathan Shay described post traumatic stress disorder as the result of the betrayal of *thémis*, a Greek word that means "divine law." *Thémis* implies a way the universe is supposed to function, a sense of justice and right. Having your marriage fall apart while you are away fighting for your country might destroy this sense of *thémis* and could explain the symptoms of the one young Marine, but most Soldiers, Sailors, Airmen, and Marines that I treated for PTSD did not feel that their country or their families had let them down. To the contrary, America seemed unified in their support of the troops. There was controversy about the wars themselves, but even those who most vehemently opposed the invasions of Iraq or Afghanistan were not calling us baby killers. Nevertheless, despite social circumstances much different from those in Vietnam, Service Members were still developing psychological difficulties.

It is interesting how many times in history PTSD had been "discovered" and renamed. Observers in each era often thought the condition was caused by a particular, new stress. In the mid-1800s, the British surgeon Earl de Grey attributed the condition of *soldier's heart*, a racing heartbeat and anxiety noticed in war Veterans, to the heavy weight of military equipment carried by English soldiers. A few years later, Jacob Mendes Da Costa observed the same phenomenon in American troops in the Civil War and blamed it on the poor nutrition of Union and Confederate soldiers. In 1876, surgeon Arthur Davy saw that well-fed officers could likewise suffer and thought the pounding pulse was due to the military habit of "over-expanding the chest, [which] caused dilation of the heart, and so induced irritability."

That a unique stress might lead to unique symptoms has not completely fallen out of favor. After Operation Desert Storm, a variety of maladies were lumped together under the moniker of "Gulf War Syndrome." A host of theories have been presented to explain it, from the possibility of nerve agents to a combination of vaccines and antimalarial drugs. That stress universally contributes to postwar syndromes does not mean that the type of physical or mental stress cannot influence the manner or frequency by which such symptoms present.

More soldiers were killed and wounded in World War I than in any other conflict in history. In a single battle, the Battle of the Somme, the British suffered almost half a million casualties. Half of these were psychological. The mental collapse was felt to be due to damage to the nervous system from the shock wave of heavy artillery. The malady was termed *shell shock*. The term fell into disfavor when it was discovered that the same symptoms could befall victims whose horror did not involve explosions.

The prevalence of improvised explosive devices (IEDs) in Iraq revived the idea, if not the terminology, of shell shock. As I was stationed in Iraq, I reviewed several hundred records from my home institution. I was not terribly surprised to find that PTSD symptoms were more prevalent in those who had been blown up than in those who were shot. When the body is rattled, the mind becomes vulnerable.

In Fallujah, we treated a string of IED survivors. I asked our chief ER physician and three-war veteran, Captain Cogar, what he thought about the effects of blast on the brain.

"I'm not sure," he said. "Traumatic brain injury does seem to be particularly prevalent now. There was a theory postulated that the body armor we are using may transmit more of the blast to the brain. It may be that because the newer armor improves survivability overall, that individuals who otherwise would have died live on with brain injuries. The bombs are also bigger than they were in older wars."

"How else do you think our current wars are different?" I asked.

"It's the longest war we have ever fought with an all-volunteer force," he pointed out. "In Vietnam, we did have a few guys who did three tours, but now we have people who have done four, even five tours. We had one sniper who was seen for shrapnel wounds who had 150 confirmed kills. I didn't even ask him how many times he had been shot at."

"Well, it's not exactly an all-volunteer force," I noted. "I seem to have had an extraordinary number of patients in my office who were involuntarily recalled."

"The burden falls on the few," said the captain. "It is a smaller group now. In Vietnam, Korea, and most of all World War II, everyone was involved. Even if you weren't serving, you knew your number could come up. During World War II, it would have been hard to find a person in America who did not personally know a Soldier who had died or been wounded in the war. It gave a strong incentive to stay informed and on top of the news. Even the atrocities of war were shared. *Life* magazine ran a picture of a decapitated Japanese head that had been taken as a trophy during the Battle of Guadalcanal. There were a few protesting letters, but a picture of a mistreated cat in the same issue generated twice as many complaints. The editors responded to the protests by reminding people that it is more dangerous to forget the inhumanity of war than to be shocked by reminders. I'm not saying that this kind of morality was good, and I don't disagree with Commander Moser that we are better supported now than we were in Vietnam. But all the cheerleading in the world doesn't make up for the fact that, while America goes about its business, the current crop of Soldiers and Marines have been out in the field for an awfully long time. It's isolating and exhausting."

I thought about some of my patients and how hard it was for them to share their experiences with friends and family members. A phrase I had gotten used to hearing was, "People ask, but they don't really want to know." Could that sense of isolation be making things worse for the most recent Veterans? Statistics show that, in general, Service Members who have a strong sense of connection and camaraderie do better than those who feel isolated. When you are part of a professional rather than an all-inclusive military, it is easy to feel set apart from the rest of the world. The country can at times forget that people are dying every day.

When Veterans return, it can be surreal to find that news is focused on gas prices and celebrity scandals when their comrades have bled and died. The support is good, but when the world seems to go on about its business, support can seem like lip service.

The War on Terror was also the ultimate multifront conflict. Two wars raged simultaneously in the deserts and marshes of Iraq and in the mountains and barren terrain of Afghanistan. Both these nations contained hundreds of smaller enclaves and conflicts within them, and terrorism wasn't confined to these countries. The enemy held allegiance to no flag. The shifting nature of the war or wars meant that it was difficult to nail down where or why the fighting was going on. Our troops could be asked to fight almost anywhere in the world at any time.

"It's difficult to think of the current conflict in terms of traditional war or counterinsurgency," Captain Cogar spoke again. "We do a great job of training our Service Members to maneuver and fight the enemy, but how do you train someone to be hit when you can't shoot back? You ride along in the truck, and bam, you are blown up by something that is completely out of your control."

"It's not just blasts, though," Commander Moser added. "We still have people out there who are doing traditional counterinsurgency work." He was referring largely to his SEAL brethren and other Special Operations troops. "But even as a counterinsurgency, there are still issues that make this war different."

"How about the fact that it is the first war with women on the front lines?" chimed in Dr. Colleen Barnum, herself the first woman to serve as an operational stress control officer, a psychologist embedded directly with frontline combat units.

I offered up the idea of how unusual it was that we had Service Members who were constantly cycling between home and war. They built up home lives each time, only to have to leave them behind again. In meeting with individuals who had come through these cycles, I was also struck by the diversity of their experiences.

For many in the initial invasion, the war had been traditional air, tank, and trench warfare. Bullets came from the direction that you expected. The enemy was in uniform. At the same time, this was the period of greatest physical hardship. Troops slept in trenches, sometimes next to corpses. Planes were shot down. Tanks could still be destroyed. Troops went without food or water for days. Communication with loved ones, or even showering, were luxuries that came only after months of hardship.

Then came a period of brief elation, of victory, followed by a sense of betrayal on both sides. The bad guys no longer wore uniforms to identify themselves. The people who had danced in the streets and overturned statues of Saddam Hussein found that their country was torn apart. Our troops, who felt they had fought and died for the freedom of this country, found the Iraqis not grateful, but murderers in our midst. Americans were burned alive and their bodies strung up in the city outside our camp.

The Battle of Fallujah ensued. Areas once conquered had to be retaken, and at great cost. Pocked cement and a plaque marked the spot outside the door to our hospital where a mortar round landed, killing a physician who was preparing to go home. Here, in what was called Operation Iraqi Freedom II, U.S. troops faced the highest casualty rates of the war.

Then came disillusionment. The story of the Vietnam conflict seemed to be playing itself out again. As in Vietnam, the U.S. military had won every battle but was losing the war. The weapons of mass destruction did not appear. Scandals such as Abu Ghraib divided military and civilian feelings about our own morality. With multiple deployments, troops were becoming exhausted. New types of stress set in.

I arrived in Iraq at a time of renaissance. The surge and Anbar Awakening had improved conditions. In our camp, we had modern plumbing, air conditioners, and all the ice cream we could eat. Most important, fewer people were dying. The lower casualty rates meant that our medical group was to be only half the size of the unit we replaced.

Although the danger had lessened, that did not mean it did not exist. The previous medical group had managed to go its entire seven-month deployment without treating a combat injury, but, in our first week in Iraq, a Marine with shrapnel in his neck was rushed to our ER. Worse would soon follow. Tragedy, although it occurred less often now, was still present. In ways, it could be even harder on the unlucky few, because it was both unexpected and unshared.

Current improvements in the country did not make the past go away. As I quickly discovered, many of the troops in Iraq during my deployment were dealing with the problems of earlier battles. They were becoming exhausted. The surge had improved conditions but also meant that troops were in the field more often. The prospect of additional strain from Iran and other hot spots meant that many Service Members felt they might never escape the cycle of battle. In and out of the valley of death they went, and there was nothing in textbooks about what to do with an individual who came to combat already diagnosed with PTSD.

Considering all the ways in which stress presented in Iraq, one remarkable fact was that business at the mental health clinics remained stable no matter what. We never experienced the waves of panicked soldiers we feared might overwhelm the system, nor did the war ever become something that was easy to accept.

"War is always hard," said one of my patients, who was in his fifth deployment. "There is no way around that. I think it is a little better now. This time, you were there to ask me how I was doing."

# 4

# Mind and Brain

THE space in the magnetic resonance imager was the size of a coffin. Petty Officer Trowel had been trapped under machinery before. He had been in a Humvee turnover after an IED blast, so he wasn't fond of small spaces. We were both safely in the United States at this point, but I knew that, for Trowel, the experience might bring up unpleasant flashbacks.

Trowel hesitated for only a moment. "Let's do it," he said.

The platform moved forward, carrying the man into the machine. I stayed in the viewing area, about a hundred feet away. Being near the scan was not inherently dangerous, but unlike Trowel, I had not been carefully searched for metal. As you approached the powerful electro magnets of the MRI, the force on a pen or a tie-clip would be enough to convert these innocuous items into deadly projectiles.

In the absence of any iron or steel with which to play havoc, the magnetic force instead started to align and stimulate subatomic particles in Trowel's brain. While not altering or repairing any of the damage that might lie therein, this magnetic resonance did allow a digital picture to take form. The gray images started to appear on the computer screen in the MRI reading room.

"Everything looks pretty normal," said the duty radiologist. "No indications of volume loss or mass effect. He had a head injury?"

"Yes, from an IED blast. He also has a bad case of PTSD," I added.

"Well, there's nothing I can see here." The radiologist practically rolled his eyes. The unspoken context was that once again I was wasting his time.

"How's the volume of the hippocampus?"

"It's slightly smaller than average, but nothing out of the normal range."

"Yeah, but he was better than normal."

Trowel had been an independent duty corpsman assigned with the Marines. *Corpsman* is the Navy term for a medic. The best and most senior corpsmen are sometimes given additional training and allowed to operate independently of their physician supervisors. They are called "Doc" by the units with which they travel, and although their formal training is brief, they are faced with situations that would overwhelm the most experienced physicians. They have to be sharp.

Since the accident, Trowel's memory had not been what it once was. He forgot names, directions, what medications he had prescribed to members of his unit. For anyone else, this might not have been serious. Everyone forgets his car keys once in a while. Trowel had compensated the way most of us do. He wrote things down, kept lists. He was still a good health care provider and well loved by the Marines whose care he was charged with. But it bothered him. Prior to his accident, Trowel had prided himself on having an almost photographic recall. He didn't anymore, and he wanted to know why.

The area of the brain that the radiologist and I were discussing, the hippocampus, is a seahorse-shaped structure deep in the cortex. It controls how new memories are laid down. In evolutionary terms, it is one of the oldest parts of the mammalian brain, having very similar makeup regardless of whether you are looking at mice, at monkeys, or at men. Unfortunately, ancient creatures had less interest in defending their brains than other body parts. This legacy has left us with a memory control area that is vulnerable to damage from strokes, repeated seizures, head trauma, or simple aging. Many people beyond a certain age can testify that, although general reasoning remains sharp throughout life, "senior moments," in which a person is left searching for the most recent details of life, become more common as years go on.

Stress can greatly accelerate brain aging. It is a curiosity of design that the most common neurotransmitter in the brain, glutamate, the chemical that allows different brain cells in the hippocampus to communicate, is actually toxic to those same cells. It takes a great deal of energy to defend the brain cells against their own dangerous signals. During periods of stress, as more and more urgent signals come in, transmission of glutamate goes up. Simultaneously, the body starts shifting defense resources to other areas that ancient creatures considered more vital. This leaves the hippocampus vulnerable.

Stress-related processes may cause traumatic memories to be physiologically "burned in" deeper than other events and helps explain why it is so much harder to forget a traumatic event or to overlay that event with other, happier recollections. This remains unproved. What is known for sure is that if a rat is exposed to stress-equivalent levels of certain hormones, its hippocampus and memory will fail much faster than they otherwise would. Similarly, in the wild, monkeys that live in high-stress situations experience hippocampal damage at much higher rates than primates that lead seemingly placid lives. Finally, we know that, on average, people with PTSD have a smaller hippocampus than those blessed with health.

So why couldn't we tell if Trowel had PTSD by looking at his hippocampus? Well, it turns out that, as with most things in the brain, humans are much more complex than white mice. In lab animals, generations of inbreeding has made every individual almost identical to every other. If a brain structure in one mouse is smaller than average, it is reasonable to assume that something has gone wrong. Furthermore, since they are raised in completely controlled conditions, it is relatively simple to see what factors are different between the small-brained animal and his large-brained twin. We humans are much more varied. It is possible, given his better-than-average memory, that Trowel had once had a larger hippocampus, but looking at his brain now, all we could say was that it was within the normal range.

Detecting PTSD by looking at brain volume is further confused by difficulties sorting out cause and effect. To get around the problem of human variation, scientists have examined the brains of identical twins. They looked at pairs in which one brother suffered PTSD and the other did not. The assumption of this study was that the healthy twin would provide the ideal comparison, showing what the hippocampus of the PTSD patient should have looked like if war had never taken its toll. The confusing finding was that both twins had a hippocampus that was smaller than average. This left scientists with a quandary. Which came first, the small hippocampus that increased the risk for PTSD or the PTSD that damaged the hippocampus and made it smaller?

Also, other studies revealed different areas of the brain that appeared to be more consistently malfunctioning within people with PTSD. Focus shifted to neural structures, such as the *anterior cingulate*, the *pregenual anterior cingulate cortex*, the *frontal cortex*, and an area of the brain where the tissues fold in on themselves called the *insula*. Why would these areas be involved in PTSD? Was the finding of a smaller-than-average hippocampus in Trowel important at all or only a normal variation?

"It's at least reassuring to know that my brain is still there," the corpsman said as he climbed out of the machine. "I guess I shouldn't have expected a clean picture of it with 'PTSD-here' stamped on it."

"Sometimes the scans don't tell us what you have, but it is just as important to know what isn't causing your symptoms." I tried to stay positive. "You don't have a brain tumor. You didn't burst a blood vessel when you hit your head during the explosion. It's good news that we didn't see anything wrong."

"I know, but proof would be nice. I had a disability hearing last week, and the guy doing it asked me how I knew I had post traumatic stress disorder."

"What did you tell him?"

"I said you told me that was my diagnosis, Dr. McLay."

"And he asked how *I* knew this is what happened, right?"

"You got it."

"And then because I made the diagnosis by listening to what you told me, you wondered if what he was really asking was if you had been lying about your symptoms all along?"

"I take it you've had guys go through this before, Dr. McLay."

"Yes. It is difficult. Sometimes the more serious brain injuries can actually be easier on a patient because there is a lesion we can show on a scan to prove that it is there. With mild traumatic brain injury, we can't see the physical damage unless we cut apart your brain. For PTSD, it is even more difficult. We know that stress damages the brain, and in cases like yours where there has been an impact, the brain is even more susceptible to that damage. What is software and what is hardware can be hard to sort out. There are all kinds of potential causes for this."

"But one of those is faking?" Trowel said, still obviously pondering the absence of any particular finding on his scan.

"That is true for many medical diagnoses, not just PTSD or TBI. The only way I know if a person has pain is what they tell me. Ninety percent of diagnosis is based on the patient's story. But, I know it's frustrating," I answered, "for everyone."

As easy as it can be to be angry with the faceless bureaucrat who questioned Trowel's claim, I could sympathize with the bureaucrat's plight, too. People do lie, both about their combat record and their symptoms. The reasons I believed Trowel suffered from PTSD were not because of lab tests, brain scans, or special tricks of the medical trade. It was simply that Trowel had no motivation to make things up. More important, the reports from friends and family members matched what he had told me himself. Either it was a giant conspiracy on the part of a large group of people coached in the particular symptoms of PTSD, or Trowel was what he seemed—an honest man with an honest problem.

I believed Trowel had PTSD because I had spent hours and days with the man. The bureaucrat did not have this luxury. He had no way of knowing whether Trowel was an honest man or if I was a competent physician making the diagnosis. Even if he did trust my judgment, he surely would know that, as a human, I'm fallible. I've been wrong before. When you only have a few moments to make a very expensive decision, it is easier to trust a machine. Unfortunately, for the bureaucrat, the machines are simply not that good yet.

The technology of current brain scanning was not at the level where we could detect the changes that occur in most PTSD cases, but newer options are on the horizon. Most MRI machines are similar to the one through which Trowel had traveled. They give a picture of what the brain looks like but say nothing about how it is being used. The picture would look the same if Trowel were sleeping, awake and thinking about pleasant memories, or having the worst PTSD flashback of his life. A technology called *functional* MRI, however, has begun to allow us to examine brain structure and brain activity.

Functional MRI, or fMRI, is still in its infancy. Only a few large hospitals have them, and even then they are usually used as a research tool and not to make a clinical diagnosis. The steady brain buzz makes it too difficult to distinguish one mode of thinking from another. It's like trying to identify a particular image when 99 percent of the picture is static. Despite this, scientists have been able to pick up changes in the brains of those with PTSD.

A small, almond-shaped section of brain lights up brightly. This area is called the amygdale. It sits at the tail of the hippocampus and seems to be involved in attaching the emotional content to memories. At least one research study found overactivity in the amygdale of 75 percent of patients with PTSD. Activity in another section of brain, called *Broca's area*, is less consistent in its changes but, in general, seems to be underactive. This quiet section of a PTSD patient's brain is normally responsible for language and naming. The other areas of the brain already mentioned, the cingulate cortex, the frontal area, and so on, may also be different.

Although this type of brain scan may one day be used to identify individuals with PTSD, it does little to help with the chicken-or-egg issue. Is the amygdale more active because an individual has painful emotions, or are their emotions so painful because their amygdale is overactive? Is the silence in Broca's area the cause or effect of Trowel's inability to describe those painful emotions? Is there really a difference?

A key philosophical advance of modern neuroscience is that brain is mind. Separating PTSD symptoms from their biology is as artificial a distinction as trying to figure out whether a video game image is caused by the computer program or the computer chip. They work, or fail, together.

None of this helped Trowel because we didn't have an fMRI.

"What else ya got?" Trowel asked as we reviewed the unremarkable looking images of his brain together.

"To detect PTSD," I shrugged, "not a whole lot right now." There were other variants of brain imaging besides MRI: positron emission tomography (PET), computed tomography (CT or CAT scan), single photon emission computed tomography (SPECT), three-dimensional electroencephalography (3D-EEG), magnetoencephalography (MEG), and so on. Although the technology at the time varied, the results were unlikely to do so. Any way you looked at it, we could show that populations were different, but identifying what exactly was or was not wrong in Trowel's brain would elude us.*

"What about serotonin?" he said. "Those commercials on TV say that is what is wrong with me. I don't have enough, and that's why I'm depressed and have PTSD."

"Maybe," I said, "but the only way to tell for sure would be to take out your brain, put it in a blender, and run it for chemical analysis."

"Well, my wife did say I never use it anyway."

"Sorry, Sailor, your brain is still government property, and Navy regulations require you to store it properly within your skull."

Trowel and I talked more about serotonin as we walked. Thanks to advertising on behalf of antidepressants that increase this brain biochemical—brands such as Prozac, Paxil, Zoloft, Celexa, and Lexapro—serotonin had become a household name.

The truth is that it has been remarkably difficult to demonstrate that serotonin is actually low in PTSD patients. It is much more common to see alterations of other hormones and biochemicals: noradrenaline is up, testosterone is low, cortisol is up and then down. The whole brain soup is different. Much of the reason scientists focus so much on serotonin is simply that the medications that increase the biochemical seem to alleviate PTSD symptoms.

This is good news for patients, but it is really not much in the way of evidence. No one thinks that low levels of penicillin are involved in the origin of syphilis because the antibiotic works against the disease. Serotonin meds might be working in many other ways rather than by increasing a chemical that is low. Antidepressants have been shown, at

---

* At the time of Trowel's scan, there was no imaging technology that could detect PTSD in individuals. Subsequently, several research groups, including programs we worked with, developed scans that may be able to see the individual changes in PTSD and traumatic brain injury. A clinical interview, however, is still the gold standard for identifying the condition.

least in test tubes, to help brain cells regenerate. And, as Peter Kramer famously described in *Listening to Prozac*, they have been thought of as a way of enacting a "global reset for the brain" rather than fixing a specific deficit.

"To give the serotonin people proper credit," I told Trowel, "I think that it actually is involved. We do have evidence that the system is perturbed, but it is a gross oversimplification to say that one thing is missing, and all we have to do is replace it."

Trowel shrugged at the distinction. "Up, down, perturbed, whatever you want to say about it, is there really no way to test it in me that doesn't involve my brain in a jar?"

"Well, you can see the breakdown products of serotonin in the urine, but we aren't sure that relates to levels in the brain. We can also do procedures like a spinal tap to look at the fluid that bathes the brain, but I don't think it's worth the pain or the risk for a test that doesn't tell us much. And of course there is that genetics study I told you about."

Several months earlier, Naval Medical Center had become involved with research started by Dr. Dewleen Baker at the San Diego VA hospital. She had intriguing evidence that indicated that people with a particular variation of a gene involved in moving serotonin in and out of cells might be at higher risk for PTSD. She was looking to confirm this by comparing the DNA of combat Veterans. Genetic screening is expensive but fairly straightforward to do. All you need is a tiny blood sample. Because of the research grant, we could easily get Trowel tested. He would be doing science and me a favor by getting the test. He looked uncomfortable, though, and I didn't want to push him.

Trowel's father had also suffered from PTSD, in that case from the Vietnam War. It is an uncomfortable idea to think that we could be born ill-fated. It can be worse still to blame it on the bloodline of a beloved parent. Although many of us hope that genetics will open the pathways to new treatments in mental health, it is still highly controversial. Gene therapy for PTSD or any psychiatric disorder is decades away at best; so, for now, the genes you are born with are the ones you have for life. We might test him, but if we did, he had a lot to lose and little to gain.

"Even if you had the gene, it doesn't mean that was the cause," I said. "Sometimes there are identical twins in combat, and one of them gets PTSD, and the other doesn't. We don't really know why."

"It's complicated. That seems to be what you say about all of it."

I nodded. "Well, it is. We like straightforward and simple explanations, but this is a brain disease. The brain is the most complex thing we know of in the entire universe. There are more cells in your brain than there are stars in the Milky Way. There are a quadrillion cell connections; that's a thousand trillion. Each of those connections may contain a variety of different neurotransmitters, and each of those neurotransmitters may act differently, depending on the molecules sitting on the next neuron in line. So dang right, it's complicated."

He laughed, a good sign. "A thousand trillion, huh? Give it a few years, and the national debt will outstrip it."

"Maybe, but hopefully, by then we'll have a cure."

He suddenly turned serious. "I don't think I can wait that long, Dr. McLay."

I hoped he didn't have to. "Why don't we go talk about a few different types of treatments," I said. "I still don't know how aspirin works, but it will cure a headache."

"It just so happens that I have a headache."

"Well, at least I can do one thing useful today, then. If we're lucky it will be two."

He agreed. Hope for two.

# 5

# The Forgotten War

WHAT happened in Afghanistan?" I asked the young man sitting in my office in Fallujah, Iraq.

"I don't know," said Corporal Winnow. "I just remember that it was different. It was colder. There were mountains. I was closer to people."

"So do any of those details seem prevalent in your dreams?"

"I'm not sure," he said. "It is hard to remember."

Corporal Winnow had come to me complaining of nightmares. They were an illogical cacophony of images, but one dream had stuck in his mind and recurred night after night. A man in a headscarf was shooting with an AK-47. The man was closing in on two American Marines from behind, but they seemed oblivious to his presence. Corporal Winnow was in a better position to return fire, but he found himself unable to move or to call out. He awoke each night from this dream, shaking and dreading any return to slumber.

Psychiatrists do not, as a whole, make as much of dreams as in the time of Freud and Jung. The "royal road to the unconscious," as Freud called dreams, turns out to be often unnavigable. If dreams do, as a whole, have particular meaning, that meaning has so far escaped modern science. In the case of PTSD, however, there seems to be an obvious explanation. Particularly powerful thoughts are so pervasive in the brain that they come out in conscious memory as well as in dreams and flash-backs. By confronting the original event in waking life, the nightmares can be made to recede.

The problem for Corporal Winnow was that it was not entirely clear what his dreams were about. He had been through three military deployments, two to Iraq and one to Afghanistan, but claimed to have not been particularly traumatized during any of them. His memories of both his previous two deployments were fuzzy. A failure to remember aspects of a traumatic event can be a symptom of PTSD. However, there are other, more benign explanations for poor memory or bad dreams. He had a mortgage to pay and felt under attack by the banks. Perhaps the dreams were just a way of expressing such anxiety. It is difficult to nail down exactly whether something is PTSD if you don't even remember what happened.

"We definitely saw gruesome things in Afghanistan," the corporal explained. "I can't remember them all, but I do remember a bus that was blown up by a roadside bomb. I was part of the team that had to pick up the pieces—hands, heads. A couple of them you could tell were kids. That was horrible, but there is nothing in the dream like that."

"The man in the dream is shooting at you," I said. "You did experience small-arms fire on all your deployments?"

"A few times, yes, but nothing so close. The snipers in both places know to run away before we can figure out where they are and return fire."

The tactics employed by the enemy in these events could have easily occurred in either country. The Iraqi army, if poorly trained, was at one time still reasonably well equipped and modern. The Republican Guard was overcome with classic use of combined arms. In Afghanistan, any weapon larger than a man was long ago destroyed by the Soviets and years of tribal warfare. Now, battles in both countries were dominated by improvised explosive devices, the Kalashnikov, hit and run, and indiscriminate bursts of terror.

It was telling of the similarities between the two conflicts that Winnow could not even identify the faction of the shooter. Both countries are marked by a dizzying array of tribal, ethnic, and religious divisions that make it difficult to keep track of who is fighting whom. Both places also had a number of outsiders come into the country to add to the chaos. The existence of al-Qaeda in Iraq before the war is questionable, but there was no doubt that it was there after the war started. What Winnow would have known for sure if he were under attack by such individuals is that they were fanatically devoted to killing him.

"How do you remember feeling in the dream?" I asked. "Were you scared?"

"I was," he said, "which is odd, because in the real firefights I have been in, I don't remember feeling that way. Especially here in Iraq, we usually outgun the insurgents by so much that it seems ridiculous. The last time we went out on patrol, there was a convoy of eight trucks filled with Marines, a couple of light-armored reconnaissance vehicles, and a tank. Some idiot insurgent tried to throw a grenade at the lead vehicle. Other than hearing a couple of fifty cals go off, I wouldn't have even known we were attacked."

"But in Afghanistan you weren't that protected?" I asked.

"No. It is hard to use heavy vehicles in the mountains. Even in the cities, we didn't go out as much. The country is bigger, so there's more territory to cover, and fewer people to cover it. Here, we are usually working right alongside the Iraqi police, but in Afghanistan, we let the locals do most of the policing and only went after the Taliban and al-Qaeda strongholds when we found them."

Finding such forces in Afghanistan and the borderland regions of Pakistan was a difficult task. America had been involved in Afghanistan for two years longer than we had been in Iraq, but in some ways, the progress had been more nebulous. In Iraq, there clearly had been a strong central government under Saddam Hussein. Saying that anyone had ever truly ruled Afghanistan was a dubious claim.

The territory that is now Afghanistan has been overrun by empires from the Persians, to Alexander the Great, the Indians, the Islamic Caliphate, the Mongols, the British, the Russians, and more. It has been called the graveyard of empires, but it has also been the gateway between them. So many cultures have embedded themselves in Afghanistan that it makes Iraq look homogeneous by comparison. The shape of modern Afghanistan was first carved out in the eighteenth century by the Durrani Empire, which created the capital cities of Kandahar and Kabul. In the wake of World War I, the territory became a buffer state between the British and Russian empires. Although it formally had its own king, or emir, Afghanistan remained largely under British control until the Third Anglo-Afghan War, when the country gained independence in 1919. If attempting to hold on to Afghanistan had damaged the British Empire, it did far worse to the Soviets after their invasion in 1978.

The Soviet Army was noted for its ruthless militarism. Between six hundred thousand and two million Afghan civilians were killed during the Soviet occupation. With billions of dollars in covert military aid from the United States, the people and the landscape of Afghanistan drove back the largest army in the world. This is cited as a failure of pure force in subduing a hostile territory. What is perhaps less well known is how this area of the world also turned back more subtle means of persuasion. The left-wing columnist and cartoonist Ted Rall noted that when traveling in the region he was surprised to find that the Soviets had tried to respect the Afghan people and their culture. Despite these attempted courtesies, the foreigners still had to be driven out and killed simply because they were foreigners.

"Afghans are the friendliest people in the world, and the most fanatical," my patient explained. "When I first came to Afghanistan, I was convinced we were going to get bin Laden and be out in a few months. We never counted on how much the people would protect him."

There is a long-standing tradition of hospitality in Afghan culture. One simply does not turn one's guest over to the invader, even if he is a mass murderer and there is a multi-million-dollar price on his head. In Iraq, the opposing forces proved much more susceptible to persuasion.

"Here in Iraq, some of the same people we were shooting at last time are now the police chiefs," explained Corporal Winnow. "It's kind of messed up. I know it is a good thing that there is progress, that there is something to work toward. But it is hard to know who to trust. In Afghanistan, it was more straightforward. There were uneducated conscripts, but, among the faction leaders, the people who hated us, really, really hated us. At least you knew who to shoot at, even if we didn't know where to find them."

Unlike Iraq, in Afghanistan there was little to fight over except ideology. Iraq has great oil reserves, fertile river basins, and palaces and other cultural landmarks. By contrast, Afghanistan is landlocked, frequently subject to earthquakes, and has a terrain mixed between freezing mountains and the Sistan Basin, one of the driest regions on earth. War and deliberate vandalism destroyed most of Afghanistan's cultural artifacts. Most infamously, the one-thousand-five-hundred-year-old giant carvings of Buddha at Bamiyan were purposefully destroyed by the government in 2001. Although there may be vast mineral reserves in the southeast and north, these remain untapped because of a lack of technological and skilled human resources. The country's main export to the world is opium.

From 1996 until the NATO-led invasion in 2001, most of Afghanistan was ruled by the Taliban. The word *Taliban* means "student," and many of its leaders were teachers from the Sunni Madrasah religious schools. The remainder were mostly conventional warlords from the mountainous Pashtun regions of southern and western Afghanistan. Although Pashtun-speaking people account for only a little over half of the population, they ended up in control of about 90 percent of the country. The Taliban's rule was marked by draconian laws drawn from a mixture of Islamic scriptures, Sharia law, and Pashtun tribal codes. This was initially welcomed throughout most of Afghanistan because of the level of corruption and crime that it was replacing. The Taliban's extreme antimodernism, along with persecution of other ethnic groups, soon degraded its popularity. The Taliban government ended up allied, often against its own people, with other radical Sunni Muslim groups such as al-Qaeda. Afghanistan, already filled with war-hardened veterans of the Soviet and civil wars, became an ideal training ground for terrorists such as those who launched the attacks on September 11, 2011.

"I'll give the Afghanis this," said Corporal Winnow. "They do know how to fight. Here in Iraq, we are always the ones on the offensive, but just last week the Taliban overran a French base in Afghanistan."

"Do you think that affected you differently?" I asked. "Were you afraid of being overrun?"

"Me? No. There was a higher chance of being killed here in Iraq by indirect fire than of being overrun in Afghanistan. I don't think I even thought about it at the time. If we had gone after the strongholds in the mountains, that would have been dangerous, but at the time, I felt safer there than here in Iraq.* We were a tighter group in Afghanistan, so that kept my mind off the bad memories."

"Do you think the nightmares are about Afghanistan?"

"It's possible. But I didn't have the nightmares there."

"It is not uncommon in PTSD that symptoms don't show up until after the deployment is over. These nightmares could have started with Afghanistan and only surfaced because of a reminder you encountered here. Do you feel that you left Afghanistan changed?"

"Your first war experience always changes you," he said. "I know I had all the classic PTSD stuff when I first came home, but it went away after a couple of weeks. I thought I was doing fine. I still think that it's my mortgage that's stressing me the most."

"And you are sure that now you are not trying to avoid thinking or feeling about the things that happened in your earlier deployments? You aren't more angry, or jumpy, or on your guard?"

"Not really, no. I know that you think this might be related to the war, Doc, but other than the nightmares themselves I can't think of anything that is stressing me out except my mortgage. That, and I'm worried if I'll be worse once I go home."

It was difficult to predict what would happen to Winnow once he left Iraq. Medical prediction is based on recognizing particular patterns of symptoms and knowing how others with that pattern responded in the past. Like many of the patients I saw in Iraq, however, his symptoms didn't fit into a particular niche. He had PTSD-like symptoms but not a classic spectrum of problems. Could a person even have *post* traumatic stress disorder if he or she was still inside the conflict? Did it matter that his most traumatic experiences occurred in a different combat zone? His nightmares seemed to be linked to combat somehow, but which combat, which war? If the problems resulted from Afghanistan instead of Iraq, did that make a difference? These were all questions for which I did not have clear answers. There was one question to which I did have a better response, however.

"So what do we do now, Doc?" Winnow asked.

---

* Such an offensive occurred in 2010, when Forces of the American-allied coalition pushed into Taliban-occupied strongholds.

"We make sure you get better," I said. "Your condition isn't text-book, so there is going to be guesswork and mutual give-and-take as we work together, but I am convinced that you don't have any symptoms or problems that can't be improved dramatically. First, we will work together more to see if we can figure out where these symptoms come from. It is helpful to have a sense of that, but even if we don't figure that out, it doesn't mean we can't do anything. There are basic rules that we have learned over the years about what does and does not work when dealing with traumatic experiences. We will work on using the logical part of your brain to overcome the powerful and negative emotional reactions you have had: mind over mood as some have called it. We also have medications that help particular symptoms. For example, there is a medication that can prevent nightmares. There are techniques you can learn to control your own dreams. There are also meds and therapies that can help you sleep. I am going to outline a collection of potential treatments that you might want to try. We are going to pick one, and then we will keep working together until we find what works for you. That and you might want to talk to a financial counselor about your mortgage."

Winnow laughed. "OK," he said. "I'll do that. How about you start telling me about those treatments."

# 6

# Treatment and Cure

DR. Holley waved her hand back and forth intensely in front of the confused-looking tech sergeant. The man did his best to keep his gaze on her fast-moving fingers. His eyes bounced back and forth, from left to right. It was like he was watching a tennis match played in fast forward.

"Blank out your mind," Dr. Holley instructed when the ocular gymnastics had stopped. "Good," she said after a short pause. "OK, what are you thinking about now?"

"Still about dogs," the patient explained. "Not necessarily about the ones that were shot but still about dogs."

Dr. Holley nodded in understanding. "And on a scale of one to ten, how distressing is that for you?"

"About a six."

The tech sergeant had been with a unit that was training Iraqi police. His unit adopted a litter of puppies that a junior Soldier had found in a bombed-out building. The dogs had served as mascots and were friends in a situation in which trust was hard to come by. One day, not long after an enemy sniper severely wounded one of the American trainers while he was setting up the range, the task of setting the practice area had been turned over to the Iraqis. The Americans felt that an Iraqi mole had been in on the sniper attack. The Iraqis thought that the Americans were purposefully putting the less-well-armored police in danger. The policemen would not rebel directly but devised what the Iraqis later claimed was a type of practical joke. They abducted and clubbed the American mascots, hanging them in sacks behind the targets on the range. The Americans, unknowingly, shot their own dogs. This wasn't the only image that haunted the tech sergeant, but in his mind, it served as a metaphor for all the injustice and pain he had seen.

"I want you to continue to focus on that image while you watch my fingers," Dr. Holley instructed.

The same, strange procedure was repeated. As she moved her hand back and forth, the tech sergeant's eyes danced, and Dr. Holley again asked for the image that floated into mind.

"How distressing is it now?" she asked.

"Five."

"Good, and let's go again."

The procedure continued for about forty minutes. In the last part of the session, the doctor and patient discussed how symptoms had or had not changed during the course of hand-waving. I thanked the tech sergeant for letting me sit in on his session with Dr. Holley. When he had gone, Dr. Holley explained to me what she had been doing.

"It's called EMDR," she said. "Eye movement desensitization and reprocessing. It is one of the forms of therapy that the Department of Defense recommends for PTSD. You may see the same form of treatment done with a light that goes back and forth to keep the patient's eyes moving, or occasionally, we use a type of vibrating clicker that alternately simulates the left and right hands rather than inducing eye movements."

EMDR had an inauspicious start. Francine Shapiro, a psychologist from California, was walking along thinking about distressing aspects of her life. She noticed that as she did so, her eyes moved back and forth quickly, and that at the end of doing this, she felt better. Dr. Shapiro started a school of treatment based on this personal experience and began running courses on how to perform EMDR.

Not surprisingly, much of the medical community looked on this as a sham, and Dr. Shapiro as a quack. This perception wasn't aided by the fact that rather outlandish claims were made about EMDR—that it could cure PTSD in one session, that it was a good treatment for all manner of ills, and that to perform it properly one had to receive a particular certification. That certification cost money, which had to be paid to Dr. Shapiro or to her organization. The initial studies published about EMDR were vague and poorly controlled. Also, when others tried more rigorous testing to investigate the importance of eye movements in the process, they found that the technique worked equally well when the patient kept her eyes fixed on a particular point. EMDR was often lumped in with other, so-called, power therapies, which are techniques that claim to have a special power to heal based on a trick such as tapping on parts of the body or using words in a particular way.

Sometimes, however, even poorly reasoned ideas turn out to have value. Dr. Shapiro's assumptions about why EMDR worked, or even what aspects were necessary to make it work, may have been spurious, but a lot of people who were treated with EMDR got better. Studies showed lasting improvements in the patients who had done EMDR, and work with brain scans suggested that even brain chemistry had improved. The other power therapies have not been as well tested, but many patients, and reputable therapists, say that a particular therapy has helped them.

The first step in figuring out if a treatment works is to try it out. This can help determine whether the therapy is safe and if patients will tolerate it. Just looking at things this way doesn't indicate true efficacy, however. Placebo effect is powerful. For researchers, the gold standard for determining whether a treatment works is to find a number of volunteers with a condition and then randomly split the group in half: one-half gets the real treatment and the other gets a placebo or sham procedure. If the people who got the real treatment improve more than those who receive the placebo, the treatment is said to have validity. Before giving it a definitive endorsement, researchers will also want to see the results repeated a couple of times by different groups of providers to ensure that success isn't a fluke or due to a hidden bias in a particular lab.

For PTSD treatment, this form of rigorous testing had been hard to come by. Avoidance is itself a symptom of PTSD, so finding individuals willing to put themselves under the spotlight of a research examination was difficult. Furthermore, most military patients have free health care, so there was little incentive to enroll in programs in which they might get sugar pills or fake treatment. Therefore, most PTSD research had been done with victims of other types of trauma, such as car accidents and sexual assault.

It is unclear whether what works for one type of PTSD works for other sources of trauma. In addition, complicating matters, most PTSD treatments are not pharmaceuticals but talk therapies. When testing a pill, it is relatively easy to manufacture a placebo that looks and tastes like the medication, but how do you form a placebo for psychotherapy? With EMDR, when the placebo group had been asked to only talk about their lives in general, the patients who got EMDR did better than those with the fake treatment. However, when the placebo group went through all the other steps in EMDR therapy, but kept their eyes still, both groups got better at an equal rate. Was this evidence that EMDR did or did not work?

In 2006, the US Department of Veterans Affairs commissioned some of the country's finest physicians and researchers from the Institute of Medicine (IOM) to review all available studies on post traumatic stress disorder. The findings were not encouraging. The IOM reviewed more than two thousand eight hundred different papers but found that most did not meet their standards for definitive evidence. The only treatment they clearly endorsed was exposure therapy,* the most common subtype of which is prolonged exposure. The patient tells his or her story and challenges situations in the real world that are reminiscent of the trauma. The process is repeated over and over until the fear fades. Exposure therapy had been tested in multiple settings with different types of trauma and under very standardized conditions. The therapy had been well studied, but did this mean that it was the best? The IOM did not say. It only said the evidence in other areas was too vague.

Many PTSD experts felt that the IOM had been too harsh. They went beyond even what the US Food and Drug Administration required

---

* Depending on whom you ask, virtual reality therapy is either classified as a form of exposure therapy or a new therapy based on exposure therapy. The IOM did not cite studies of virtual reality to support or refute their conclusions.

to approve a medication for treatment. Two medications had been FDA-approved for PTSD, sertraline (Zoloft) and paroxetine (Paxil), but according to the IOM, there was insufficient evidence for *any* medication. Almost everyone else agreed that medications improved but were not a cure for PTSD. Was that enough to dismiss them altogether? Standards vary on what constituted a sufficiently robust response.

In addition to the Institute of Medicine review, at least four other attempts have been made to get experts to agree on PTSD treatment. The International Society for Traumatic Stress Studies, the American Psychiatric Association, the British National Institute for Clinical Excellence, and the Department of Veterans Affairs / Department of Defense each came up with a set of guidelines. Unfortunately, all five bodies came to slightly different conclusions. There were only a few points on which they concurred.

"I know everyone agrees that exposure therapy is the most evidence-based treatment," Dr. Holley said, after her therapy session with the tech sergeant, "but this patient was so reticent that it didn't seem to be going anywhere. We need other options, and, for him, EMDR seemed to do the trick."

"What other forms of treatment have you found to be effective?" I asked.

"Well, Veterans aren't ready to open up to a civilian," she said. "But they will talk to other Vets. Dr. Slier has a group session set up. You might want to see if you can sit in."

I did, and I made my way over to the office of the tall, bearded, soft-spoken man. Dr. Slier was himself a Vietnam Veteran. He had been an enlisted grunt in the war but had left the military to get his PhD in psychology and to help his former comrades in arms. He now was using those skills to help the current generation of Service Members who had returned from Iraq and Afghanistan. Mostly, he saw patients individually, but on Tuesdays and Thursdays, he gathered them together in a circle and let them help one another.

"I'll ask the group if you can observe," he said. "I don't expect it to be a problem, but you have to get the mix right. Groups can be tricky, because one conflict can distract from everyone's progress."

I ended up joining the Thursday session. It was set up similarly to the groups that had been run on the psychiatry ward, with the session starting off with people introducing themselves and explaining why they were there. The principal difference between this group and what I had seen with John and Maria was homogeneity. Everyone in Dr. Slier's group had been shot at or blown up. That wasn't the only type of trauma that people experienced in war, of course, but Dr. Slier had handpicked this group so that, in sharing, they could realize that they weren't alone.

"I'm not afraid to say that I was scared," said a gruff-looking man in blue jeans who had introduced himself as Denzel. Some people did come to group in uniform, but, at least for this hour each day, they were encouraged to think of one another by first name rather than by rank and title. "Being scared isn't what I have a problem with. It's that we left our people behind. They say we never leave men behind, but it happens. We might bring back their bodies, but we left them there to die. We could have done more."

"We could have done more. We could have done less. We don't know what we *could* have done," chimed in a young woman in the uniform of an army specialist. She identified herself as Jan. "We only know what we did do, and what we have to do now. Beating ourselves up over the dead doesn't bring them back."

A Marine named Trung who was home from his fourth deployment nodded in agreement. He smiled at Jan, and you could tell that he liked her. In liking her, he also liked something in himself. That was, I guessed, the point.

"You seem mellow tonight, Jan," Trung said. "I guess those new pills are working out for you."

"A bit. They took long enough to kick in."

"I had the same problem with my Celexa," said a previously silent Airman called Steve. "You have to keep taking them, though. They don't work if you don't take them."

Nods went around the room. It was encouraging to see that the group listened to one another, even if they didn't always listen to their physician when I gave the same advice. The Celexa, or citalopram, that Trung had mentioned was another selective serotonin reuptake inhibitor (SSRI), the same class of medication as Zoloft, Paxil, Prozac, Luvox, and Lexapro. Only two of these brands had gone through the formal FDA process to get approved for the treatment of PTSD, but most doctors thought of these medications as similar. They worked slowly, taking six to eight weeks for people to notice any sort of difference and usually requiring six to twelve months of treatment if any lasting changes were to be effected. Unfortunately, side effects tended to kick in before the benefits, so patients often gave up early. The benefits were modest, so different scientists disagreed whether the risks were worth the benefits. Personally, I thought they were worth a shot. The medications sometimes took the edge off enough to allow a person to tolerate therapy. And if there were side effects, the medication could always be stopped. I wished if people were going to stop them, they would talk to me. It might have been a problem that we could have fixed.

"I liked those other pills better," said Denzel, "the ones they gave me for the nightmares. That worked right away. You should ask for those."

I guessed that he was either talking about prazosin (Minipress) or quetiapine (Seroquel). Neither had been reviewed by the FDA, but they were gaining ground as rapid solutions to particular problems. Prazosin was of a class of medication called alpha blockers, originally used for blood pressure, and then later popularized as a treatment for prostate problems. Prazosin blocked the effects of adrenaline and noradrenaline, substances that seemed to be too high in patients with PTSD. Prazosin didn't have much of an effect on the wider spectrum of symptoms of PTSD, but it did cause sleep to be dreamless, a clear boon for the nightmare-haunted patient. Unfortunately, unlike the SSRIs, prazosin was a drug that, if stopped suddenly, could hurt you. Since it was designed as a treatment for hypertension, its sudden withdrawal could result in an unhealthy spike in blood pressure.

Prazosin, although it helped with bad dreams, did little to actually induce sleep. For that, quetiapine was often the quick fix. This was much more controversial. Quetiapine is what is called a neuroleptic, or a second-generation antipsychotic. It and its sister drugs, risperidone (Risperdal), olanzapine (Zyprexa), and ziprasidone (Geodon), were tried in PTSD because the flashbacks that patients suffer in that condition were thought to be related to hallucinations experienced by individuals with diagnoses such as bipolar disorder and schizophrenia, for which the drugs were designed. The benefit of neuroleptics for flashbacks has not been well studied, but even without formal research, it is clear that they can knock people out. These drugs thus gained popularity as super sleeping pills. The problem, and reason that they are controversial, is that the side effects can be quite serious, and no one knows if they are really helpful for PTSD as a whole. A large VA study of risperidone found no overall benefit and that the medication only modestly improved symptoms of hyperarousal. Many military physicians discounted this study since it was done largely in Vietnam Veterans whose symptoms were much more entrenched, and presumably more resistant to medications than those of the younger Service Members we were seeing.

"What really worked for me," said Steve, a sailor with a fixed, angry expression, "was Xanax. But my doctor won't give it to me anymore."

Dr. Slier, previously a silent observer among the patients, chose this moment to interject. "Steve, we talked about this, and you know you have a problem with addiction to benzodiazepines, and with alcohol."

"Yeah, well that helped too," Steve insisted.

"So your life was better when you were drinking and taking these pills?"

"Well, no, but I felt better."

"Drinking made me feel better, too," agreed Denzel.

The issue seemed to divide the group. About a third of the group supported Steve and his solution of drinking and pills. Another third seemed ready to speak out against intoxicating remedies, and the remainder sat as spectators, waiting to see which way the overall tide would turn.

Dr. Slier, however, was not waiting for a popular vote. "On this one, you are going to have to trust me," he said. "People with PTSD often turn to alcohol or addictive drugs. Not all pills that make you feel good are good. Short-term gain can often mean long-term loss, and in PTSD, more people destroy their lives with alcohol than almost any other way. But this conversation on drugs and alcohol is getting off topic. We were talking about how Denzel felt guilty for leaving fellow Service Members behind. Did anyone else have that experience?"

This type of intervention was why it was important to have a mediator in the group. Support networks can be a powerful thing, but sometimes even well-meaning friends can give you bad information. Also, it is easy to get off topic or start yelling at one another. Having someone like Dr.

Slier in the room tended to keep things civil, truthful, and on track.

"We try and address misplaced guilt, and other distorted thinking," Dr. Slier explained after the group session had ended. "It is similar to what we do in individual cognitive behavioral therapy sessions, but it is helpful to hear these things from people who have actually been there."

Cognitive behavioral therapy, or CBT, is probably the most commonly used therapy by psychologists and psychiatrists today. There are several forms of CBT that have been specifically adapted for treating PTSD, most notably cognitive processing therapy, or CPT. In our department, the guru of this approach was Dr. Grossman. She was another civilian provider at Naval Medical Center San Diego. Unlike Dr. Slier, who had been brought onboard to specifically address issues of combat stress, Dr. Grossman had been at Naval Medical Center San Diego well before the wars in Iraq and Afghanistan. She had seen Service Members encounter a multitude of emotional difficulties and knew that CBT was a method that could help many if not most of them.

"Cognitive therapy is about using the logical, thinking part of your brain to take control of your emotions and actions. Mind over mood," she explained. "We all have certain lies, or cognitive distortions as we call them, ingrained in our thinking that tend to drive us toward negative emotions or behaviors. In CBT, we examine the truth or falsehood of these beliefs and learn to replace illogical or unhelpful thoughts with thoughts that help us to function."

Private First Class Ilirus later told me how cognitive therapy had helped him. He had been in Operation Phantom Fury and was in a unit in which casualties had been unusually high. He had survivor's guilt, but more than that, he felt trapped both by what he had done and what he had left undone.

"I had to kill a kid," he said. "He can't have been over twelve, but he had an AK, and he caught us by surprise as we were clearing a building. My squad had the rest of the family crouching against the wall while we searched, and all of a sudden this kid bursts into the room and opens up. A shot hit the squad leader in the face. Another bullet caught me in the chest, but luckily it hit right against the armor plate and I was just knocked down. Lance Corporal Cortez was right behind him, and he had the kid dead to rights, but he froze. Maybe he saw how young the shooter was. The Iraqi kid saw Cortez and turned and shot him too. I was still stunned but opened up. I was the SAW* gunner in the squad, so there wasn't much left of him after that. This kid, who wasn't much older than my baby brother, gets splattered all over his now screaming family.

"That scenario used to play over and over in my mind. Sometimes I would beat myself up because I killed the kid. Sometimes it was the opposite, and I felt guilty for hesitating. I had as good a chance as Cortez of getting a shot off before the kid fired, and then Cortez wouldn't have gotten hit. Other times, I was mad at our squad leader because he should have known there could have been someone else in the house and not had us grouped all together like that. Only, he was dead, so there wasn't any point at being mad at him.

"I was mad all the time, and I knew that it wasn't about the guy who got the parking space in front of me, but I refused to admit it. Dr. Grossman made me keep track of my thinking, so I saw how often I was thinking about this kid when I got angry. People told me over and over that there had been no way to win that day, but I didn't listen to them. When I came to therapy, Dr. Grossman had me diagram it all out. I wrote down the reasons that I should feel guilty, and the reasons that argued that it really wasn't my fault. She told me that there might be reasons I did need to feel guilty, and to not deny those, but to be honest about the other side too. Eventually, as I went through these exercises, put the truth down in black and white, something clicked. I started to not just hear the truth about the situation, but to believe it. The whole thing still sucks, but I can live with myself now. I don't feel like I'm living a lie.

"The therapy wasn't rocket science. There was nothing in those sessions that I didn't know already, but sometimes it takes repetition. It was kind of like riding a bicycle. It is a simple idea. You get on and peddle. But until you have practiced it over and over again, it is hard. Once you get it down, it's second nature."

As I interviewed patients who had gone through different treatments, I realized that there was no one-size-fits-all solution for PTSD. For

---

* Squad automatic weapon.

some, medication had been the largest boon. For others, it had been the personal interaction with a therapist. For still others, it was, in the end, friends, family members, and faith that pulled them through. For most, it took a combination of these things.

This is not to say that all treatment is created equal. There were things that did tend to work more often than others. As I said earlier, I don't think I saw anyone cured by medication alone. Likewise, those who came into therapy just looking for general support, or who only focused on the here-and-now, didn't tend to get better. For most, facing fears and directly confronting the source of trauma was a big part of the solution. But no treatment worked one hundred percent of the time. There clearly was still room for improvement. For the time being, however, we did have a good collection of treatments. There was trial and error in finding the right one for the right person. But for the individual who stayed focused, who showed up and was honest with his doctor or therapist about what was or was not working, there was usually light at the end of the tunnel.

It was our responsibility as doctors and researchers to make sure that light kept getting brighter.

# 7

# I Don't Believe in That Stuff

## Arguments against the Existence of PTSD

W HAT am I doing here?" I asked myself as I unpacked my sea bag inside the small, plywood office in Camp Fallujah. The room was silent, but luckily there was better counsel to be sought. My predecessor, Dr. Southern, would be staying around for another week and a half to help orient me to my surroundings and new job.

"Whatever you can," the captain answered. "There will be difficulties, though. You are familiar with the title of Wizard?"

"Yes," I nodded. "*Wizard* is what Marines call a psychiatrist."

"I thought it was flattering at first," she explained, "but it is really a bit of an insult. I guess witchdoctor was too obvious. Half the Service Members are going to think that everything we do is nonsense and voodoo. The other half is going to be afraid that you will find out a dark secret about them and have them kicked out of the military. The Wizard makes people disappear."

"Stigma is a big issue out here?" I asked.

"It's a huge problem," she explained. "It is hard enough in the rear or in civilian practice. In war, everything gets magnified. Much of the senior leadership is actually very supportive, but it only takes a few people to start a rumor. Peer pressure and self-doubt are serious problems."

"So do Service Members have the same issue if they come to medical with a broken foot?"

My question was a familiar one among psychiatrists. Mental health was often the neglected stepchild of military medicine. However, Dr. Southern surprised me by pointing out that it wasn't just the invisible wounds that were difficult to treat in theater.

"Actually, yes, Service Members do have a problem with coming to medical no matter what. Every hour a patient is in clinic means an hour that the unit is short a guard or a mechanic or a fifty-cal gunner. It is freezing at night, a hundred and forty during the day, and hard work no matter what time it is. The people who are doing the extra work while their colleague is missing tend to get grumpy while they are gone. They are going to assume malingering, even if they can't prove it. No one wants to get labeled that way."

"Has anyone just come out and told you they think PTSD is bull-sh–t?"

Dr. Southern mulled the question over for a moment. "Not in so many words," she said. "The prejudice is more subtle. Recommendations get ignored. Patients aren't brought in on time. That sort of thing."

I contemplated this issue as I wandered to lunch. A psychiatrist wasn't going to be much good to individuals who wouldn't or couldn't come into sessions. But what else could be done? The military hierarchy had already tried to persuade people that PTSD was a legitimate and treatable problem. Armed Forces Television was being broadcast on large-screen TVs around the chow hall as I ate. At least three of the commercials that appeared between the Fox News spots were devoted to the subject. Admiral Mike Mullen, the chairman of the Joint Chiefs of Staff, encouraged troops to come in for care if they needed it. Chaplain and peer counselors circulated, spreading the same message. Service Members were required to meet with a health care professional before deploying, on returning home, and three months later to ensure that all of their health care needs, including PTSD, were addressed. All this, and people still didn't know about or believe in PTSD.

There is a tendency to chalk such attitudes up to willful ignorance. It also would have been ignorant, however, not to acknowledge the other side, I realized. The core of scientific thinking is the critical examination of ideas. And to be honest, it wasn't just the grunts in the field who questioned certain aspects about PTSD. I remembered that, when I was a medical student rotating at Johns Hopkins Hospital, the chairman of psychiatry at that venerable institution had listed PTSD in a lecture about "fad diagnoses" that also included multiple personality disorder.

Perhaps the toughest academic challenge to the concept of PTSD is the idea that a trauma causes the symptoms. In almost every other diagnosis in the *Diagnostic and Statistical Manual of Mental Disorders*, no particular cause is attributed. Psychiatrists simply look for a pattern of symptoms and use that to make predictions and attempt cure. We sometimes like to theorize about biochemical imbalances or unhappy childhoods as "causative," but for the formal diagnosis, no such primary force is required.

In PTSD, this simplified method of thinking is jettisoned. The trauma is assumed to be the actual source of the disorder. This has implications for the nature of mental causation. In a life that can be filled with trauma and tragedy, how did we decide that this one event resulted in anger and sleeplessness and other events did not? We know that individuals with a history of childhood abuse have a higher likelihood of developing PTSD after combat. Is this because trauma is cumulative, and eventually someone just reaches his breaking point? Or did the combat trauma provide a focus for problems that had been lurking for a lifetime? Many of the symptoms of PTSD can occur in individuals who have never had a life-threatening trauma but who attribute their problems to a different type of experience such as the loss of a loved one or family stress. In those who do meet criteria for PTSD, 80 percent will have problems that overlap or could be explained by other psychiatric diagnoses, such as general anxiety disorder or major depression. People are, by their nature, multifaceted, and it can be hard to sort out what is and is not PTSD.

Beyond the academic arguments, that PTSD is the result of a particular event has practical implications. There is now something to blame for problems in a person's life. When the cause of disability is war, this means the government pays a pension. When money is involved, the science starts to take a backseat to politics and self-interest.

Physician and conservative pundit Sally Satel argued in a 2006 op-ed published in *Slate* magazine that symptoms of PTSD were perpetuated by the very idea of having such a diagnosis. "Once a patient receives a monthly check based on his psychiatric diagnosis, his motivation to hold a job wanes. He assumes—often incorrectly—that he can no longer work, and the longer he is unemployed, the more his confidence in his ability for future work erodes and his skills atrophy. By sitting at home on disability, he adopts a 'sick role.'"

An American Enterprise Institute conference statement from 2005 on the subject was even more blunt: "Generous Veterans Affairs entitlements for chronic PTSD may have created financial incentives for veterans to claim psychological disorders."

So it wasn't just the troops in the field who jumped to the idea of malingering when an individual presented with symptoms of PTSD. Many individuals from all walks of life felt that PTSD was something that was made up to justify a paycheck, a trip home, or a failed life. I was reminded of General Patton's response to a hospitalized Soldier with combat fatigue that he encountered in 1943.

"I can't stand the shelling," said the young Soldier.

"Goddamn coward," Patton screamed at the man and slapped him across the face.

Patton was removed from command for that outburst, and military personnel ever since have been wary of ranting too loudly against the diagnosis. Still, I knew the belief that PTSD was little more than cowardice remained entrenched in some circles, and I wanted to know more about why people felt this way. In a long-standing military tradition, I went to a senior enlisted man whom I trusted to see if he could ferret out information from the troops. I finished my meal and left the chow hall to cut across base to one of the Marines' administrative buildings.

"Gunny Grant." I offered my hand as I stepped into the wardroom of the senior noncommissioned officers. "I have a favor to ask. I'm looking for someone who doesn't believe that PTSD exists and would be willing to talk to me about it."

It had struck me that the gunnery sergeant was the perfect person to have such contacts if they existed. He was well liked up and down the ranks. A blunt man, who said what needed saying even when it was unpopular, Gunny Grant had a tendency to encourage similarly honest responses. Still, I was surprised by his answer.

"That's easy, Sir," he said. "That would be me."

"Really?" I said pulling up a chair. "But you had symptoms yourself. You said you were having nightmares every night after the Battle of Fallujah."

I had seen the gunnery sergeant for a few informal sessions when I first arrived on base. He had come by to talk to me about a couple of his Marines, and over time, these meetings turned from discussions about them to sessions about him. During sessions, he had told me about his experiences in previous combat deployments and from a childhood in a gang-infested neighborhood where violence was almost as common as it was in Iraq. He had been through some pretty horrific stuff. He never qualified for a full diagnosis of PTSD. That requires more severe symptoms and for them to last longer than a month. Still, he had seemed very psychologically minded and clearly had the experience to understand where the symptoms had come from.

Gunny shrugged. "Yeah, but the nightmares went away. I just find it hard to believe that a person can get into a state where they can't find joy in anything in life."

"So it's not just PTSD that you don't believe in, it's psychiatric diagnoses, period?"

"I'm not knocking what you do, Sir. I liked talking to you, and I think it is helpful to get a boost through things in life, but I have a hard time believing that someone could be completely disabled by their own thoughts."

"Well, how about in schizophrenia or traumatic brain injury? Do you think that people with those conditions could just suck it up?"

"That's different. There are clearly people with a few nuts and bolts missing from the brain machine."

"What if I told you that stress itself can damage the brain? That stress hormones can kill brain cells as easily as a blow to the head?"

Gunny pondered this for a moment. Many people seem to place a great deal of emphasis on the physical when it comes to brain disease. A software glitch can cause just as many problems as a hardware malfunction, but somehow the hardware error seems more real. To his credit, Gunny stuck to the functional argument.

"That may be so, Sir," he said. "But having nightmares versus someone who thinks they are talking to the devil? Those problems aren't
even in the same league."

"Maybe not," I said. "You don't see that it might be a problem, if the
nightmares and insomnia that you experienced were magnified a few
hundred times?"

The gunnery sergeant shrugged. "Maybe," he said. "But how do you
know that they actually are that bad? I know what I've been through.
My mother was shot in front of me when I was a kid. I've been in over
twenty firefights and was shelled nonstop for thirty days straight. I've had
people try to kill me on three continents, and I've seen men, women,
and children burned alive. I made it through. How do these punks who
have been shot at once say that they now can't get up and do their job in
the morning?"

"I don't disagree that they should do their jobs," I said, "but you must
realize that it isn't easy for some people."

"Life isn't easy," he said. "You just keep pushing harder."

I could see where Gunny Grant was coming from. Despite our advances in scientific knowledge, most of what we truly believe in comes
from either people we trust or personal experience. Gunny's experience
told him that you could just push through problems. Why should he
trust the word of people who seemed incapable of dealing with stresses
less severe than those he had already overcome?

If it were just a matter of mental toughness, though, one had to ask,
why did the United States still have combat fatigue in World War II? At
the beginning of that conflict, the US Army embarked on an aggressive
program to weed out individuals they felt were "psychologically unsuit-
able." A full 10 percent of those so screened were rejected from military
service. This aggressive screening process, however, did nothing to re-
duce the rates of combat-related psychological problems. The incidence
of combat fatigue in US troops was higher than in other countries that
adopted no such screening process.

Also, if as Dr. Satel had espoused, PTSD was a self-created problem,
re-enforced by payments to be disabled, one has to wonder why the
problem existed in even earlier conflicts. In World War I, both sides
were overwhelmed by psychological casualties well before they came

up with any sort of system for how to deal with them. Even when the incentives were impressively negative, PTSD persisted. The Germans tried painful electrical shocks to create an aversive reaction in those who lost their nerve in combat. The British later adopted gentler methods, but their first solution to the problem was to hang the offending soldiers for cowardice. Nevertheless, the problem continued. Negative incentives were abandoned not only for their cruelty but also because they didn't work.

Certainly, there are individuals who manufacture symptoms, either consciously or unconsciously. It is estimated that 2 percent of individuals who claimed PTSD after Vietnam had never actually been in the military. Malingering is hardly unique to PTSD, however. Back pain, migraine headaches, even epilepsy can be just as hard as psychological conditions to substantiate with physical evidence. If 2 percent of individuals lie about their symptoms, does this render everyone else's story equally suspect?

What about causality? How do we know that war caused these people's problems? On a purely intellectual level, causality is almost impossible to prove. Philosophers might argue that one does not know whether a ball falls because you open your hand to release it or, rather, if your hand opens because the ball was about to fall to the ground. There are still a few scientists who argue that smoking does not cause lung cancer. However, one tends to notice that most of these individuals work for the tobacco industry. In the case of PTSD, the bias works both ways. If Veterans groups have been the loudest voices arguing PTSD is a real cause of disability, then also those arguing the other side are often budget hawks looking to prevent increases in government payouts.

Perhaps the most infamous evidence of the political nature of arguments against PTSD came when a VA administrator in Temple, Texas, sent out an e-mail to her staff. It said, "Given that we are having more and more compensation-seeking veterans, I'd like to suggest you refrain from giving a diagnosis of PTSD."

Proving causality may be fraught with issues of bias and philosophical challenge. There are, however, certain commonsense arguments that seem to indicate that the symptoms are actually linked to the trauma. For example, why would you have nightmares of a firefight if the dreams weren't actually about that firefight? Also, although there are clearly in-dividuals who deploy to war with preexisting problems, there seem to be many more who came in highly functional and happy and left with debilitating issues. As one patient of mine put it, "My life was going swell six months ago. Now it's not. Something must have gone wrong."

Perhaps the most difficult argument to overcome for those who do not believe in PTSD is personal experience. Even by the worst estimates, only one in four people who have been through the trauma of war will come back with PTSD. Why should the other three believe the one? Scientists are still scrambling to answer why it is that certain people get PTSD and others do not. There may not be an easy answer anytime soon. Life can be quite random. Two people can eat the same foods and do the same amount of exercise and only one of them will drop dead of a heart attack. Fifty people can be exposed to the same level of radiation and only one of them develops cancer. Does this mean that we should not believe that healthy living is good for our hearts or that radiation comes with risks?

There are many reasons someone would or would not believe in PTSD. Truth is a hard thing to get to. I have always liked the philoso-pher William James's take on the subject. He said that things are true to the extent that they are useful. PTSD is a useful concept. It should not define who a person is or give anyone an excuse to fail, but it can give a pattern for recovery. If trauma had nothing to do with symptoms, then confronting trauma would not help a person to overcome her problems. But it does.

The military had many programs in place to convince people that PTSD exists and that they should come in for help. For all this, the most effective thing I saw for getting people into treatment was when a chief warrant officer stood up in front of her unit and told them she had been in psychotherapy.

"I know it is hard to admit," she said. "I know that you think that you are too tough for that to happen to you, or that if you say you have a problem people are going to think that you are weak, or flawed, or just didn't try hard enough. I thought that way too. I was wrong. People who know me know how hard I try, how hard I work, and how strong I still am. I'm up here now telling you that PTSD is real, and also that it is treatable. For those who doubt, ask those who knew me, am I the sort of person who would lie to you? Have I ever lied to you? Only I know what goes on inside my own head. Only you know what goes on inside yours. I ask you to believe me that I am telling you the truth."

I, for one, believed.

# 8

# *Some* Birthday

## Attempts to Prevent PTSD

SEPTEMBER 11 is my birthday. In 2001, when that fateful day arrived, my gift to myself was an extra fifteen minutes in bed. It was just after the clock started blaring National Public Radio at 5:45 a.m. Pacific Standard Time that an announcer broke in saying a plane had struck the World Trade Center. It didn't faze me. I imagined that the pilot of a small Cessna or other single-engine plane had foolishly flown too close to the twin behemoths. Compared with the greater questions getting older raised about my own mortality, events in New York seemed to play no important part in my life. The news was lost in the blurred edges of dreams and in preparations for work. I stepped out of bed onto the cold floor.

The normal physiological events involved in waking up in the morning in many ways are a scaled-down version of any response to stress. Thus, even though I was unruffled by the news, my sleepy brain had already started sending out hormonal and nerve signals to the other parts of the body. Stimulating hormones perked up, releasing hormones, which in turn floated in the blood down to little glands sitting just above the kidneys called the adrenals. From there, the hormone cortisol was released back into the bloodstream, which by now was moving much faster because electrochemical signals from my brain had traveled down through nerves to the heart and muscles, increasing heart rate and blood pressure. The cortisol and other hormones mobilized blood sugar, which fed hungry brain and muscle. As I moved into the shower, I might have thought it odd that the news was going on longer than expected about the smoke coming from the North Tower, but as the water struck, my body and my mind were calm and ready to start the day.

United Airlines Flight 175 hit the South Tower of the World Trade Center at 9:03 a.m., which was 6:03 a.m. on the West Coast. By then I was buttoning my uniform. The radio broadcaster seemed flustered.

"What are the odds?" I thought, still envisioning Cessnas. I'm sure that my pulse never increased a beat. I drove to work and was waved past the front gate at the military hospital without a second look. The employee parking lot was about a twenty-minute walk from the ward, so I had to get in by 6:30 if I was going to have time for a cup of coffee before the beginning of the 7:00 a.m. staff meeting.

The waiting room at the hospital held the first television set I had encountered that morning. Except that many of the employees were in military uniforms, the scene there was the same as that around any television in any workspace or gathering place in America. Everyone watched in horror. The footage did not seem real. Pulses quickened. Eyes dilated. The neuronal and endocrine events that brought me into wakefulness were themselves again awakened, and, this time, the brakes did not kick in. The news continued to get worse. The Pentagon was struck by another plane full of passengers. Many in the hospital had friends or relatives working there. The towers collapsed. The death toll increased. And at the largest military hospital in the world, a few wondered out loud if we could be considered a target.

Whenever a great tragedy occurs there is an impetus to want to do something. This is healthy. When it comes to preventing psychological trauma, however, it is not clear we know what to do.

At the hospital, the first decision that had to be made was what to do about the patients. Should we let them watch the news? Do we continue with a regular workday to enhance the sense of stability? What do we do to help comfort the individuals who were clearly already upset? Should we assume that those who aren't showing distress are just covering it up, or do we run the risk of destabilizing functional coping mechanisms if

we push too hard? How do we, as mental health workers, provide support when we may be at our wits' end?

"First, calm down and take your own pulse." Captain Impedio, the
head of inpatient psychiatry, took charge of the situation. She was not
normally a woman known for serenity, but, like many, she did what
needed doing when it needed to be done. Captain Impedio addressed
the hospital staff.

"This is a new situation for all of us, so there isn't going to be a text-
book answer. Remember, though, that much of mental health is just the
rigid application of common sense. In some cases, we might not know
what exactly to do, but we know unhealthy when we see it. Let's start by
keeping that in mind."

On that morning, thanks to television, almost every person in America
saw the same horrific scene over and over again. For all of America, it was
a traumatic event. In retrospect, however, we know that almost no one
who watched the events of that day on television suffered PTSD as a result.
Even among the residents of the attacked cities, rates of psychiatric impairment were not drastically increased except in areas directly under threat.
Residents living north of Canal Street in Manhattan would suffer PTSD
at only a third the rate of those living closer to the towers. Fear and horror were certainly there, stress hormones and physiological changes were
present, but for those unlucky enough to develop post traumatic stress,
an additional element must have been present or a positive factor missing.

Patients on our ward were allowed to keep up with the news. The
events of the day were terrible, but we figured that not knowing would
be worse. To those for whom the television footage might be too graph-
ic, we tried to explain the situation as honestly as possible. A picture
may tell a thousand words, but sometimes the words are better. If people
asked questions, we answered them. We didn't lie, but likewise we didn't
go over lurid details with those who were content to keep quiet.

"Do we want to do a debriefing for the patients or staff?" One of the
nurses asked as the day pressed on.

"No," Captain Impedio answered for all of us. "Let's just keep things
as natural as possible. I don't think a debriefing would help anything."

Debriefing, gathering in a circle and discussing our reactions after a
trauma, has worked its way into the popular culture. Jeff Bridges's movie

*Fearless* has a pretty accurate rendition of how it works. Everyone sits in a circle and goes over his or her memories and feelings of the day. A therapist, usually a stranger to members of the group, keeps things moving and prevents individuals from lashing out at one another. Such exercises have become so widespread that many institutions assume they are opening themselves up for lawsuits if they don't perform them. The problem is there is no evidence that debriefing actually works. It has been formally tested several times. People liked the debriefings, but they didn't do any better than those who got no treatment at all.

The good news is that no treatment at all is actually not that bad. In the face of a traumatic event, many individuals will have some symptoms that are similar to PTSD. Most, however, will recover quickly. These people require neither diagnosis nor treatment. We only call the problem PTSD if symptoms have persisted longer than a month and continue to cause problems in a person's life. When it comes to the early stages of treating trauma, Mom, fellowship, and apple pie are as good as anything.

The military had tried in the past to prevent PTSD. Difficult experience had taught that just pushing troops harder in war, or telling them to "snap out of it," was not effective at inducing recovery. Likewise, taking people back home and putting them on a Freudian couch did not have much better success. The middle road, normalcy, turned out to be the best approach. The military likes acronyms to explain things and had traditionally called their prevention approach "PIES," meaning Proximity, Immediacy, Expectancy, and Simplicity. In recent years, they defied the "simplicity" aspect of their own advice and expanded the acronym to BICEPS. The idea is still the same. BICEPS indicates that crisis intervention should be Brief, Immediate, conveyed through a Central contact (someone with whom the traumatized person will have an ongoing relationship), include the Expectancy of full recovery, be done Proximally (near the home or trauma environment), and emphasize the idea that treatment should be Simple.

"You'll be OK," I said over and over that day. "We are all going to be OK."

Of course, there were cases in which we knew it wasn't going to be OK. Certain factors do, as a whole, increase or decrease the chance of things going wrong. For example, we know that people who "disassociate," or lose touch with reality, during a trauma are at higher risk.

Likewise, those who turn to drugs or alcohol following stress tend to do poorly. Conversely, individuals with a strong sense of purpose, good family support, or a good ongoing relationship with a therapist or counselor have better chances of getting back to their normal lives.

"I don't know if I can take it," said John, the Vietnam vet who came to me that day. "I don't know if I can stand the idea of their being another war."

We talked for a while.

"Are you thinking about hurting yourself, John?" I asked.

John nodded. We discussed options and finally agreed that he should stay in the hospital a while longer. Time and a regular life are often the real healers. However, left alone, a person who is suicidal might not live long enough for these simple joys to work their miracles. In John's case, and for those thinking of harming themselves or others, the BICEPS principle must yield to the more universal truth that if you want to get better, you have to be alive to do so.

In these cases, a psychiatric hospital offers safety: a place with no weapons or sharp edges, a room where someone will check on you, and a nurse who will measure out one sleeping pill that night instead of allowing you to swallow twenty. Long-term treatment within the psychiatric hospital has largely gone the way of the dodo bird, but a brief period in a safe environment can often make all the difference. It's still pretty simple, but sometimes treatment means having to be away from home.

John was not alone in being questioned about suicide. As a psychiatrist, it is my job to ask that of all my patients. Surprisingly, people take this well. I've had many an individual look at me strangely when I've asked if they wanted to die, but hardly ever was the person offended. Early in my medical training, I used to worry whether I might put the idea into someone's head by asking. It does not work that way. Asking about dangerous behavior actually lowers the risk that a person will harm himself. In general, if you want to know if there is a serious problem, the simplest solution is to ask.

"What are we going to do about Mr. Wordsworth?" Lieutenant Season, our charge nurse, asked.

Mr. Wordsworth was the other case on the ward for which the BICEPS principle did not easily apply. He was our oldest patient at the time and a Pearl Harbor survivor. Unlike John, Mr. Wordsworth had come through war with psyche intact. The later years had not been so kind. He now had Alzheimer's disease. We had tried to explain the situation to him, but he was confused and scared. He had persevered through December 7 with great aplomb, but we didn't know if he would be so lucky with September 11. Sometimes it didn't seem clear whether he knew from which attack his country was suffering.

In Mr. Wordsworth's case, we decided that keeping him in the hospital was the best course. Media reports on his home television would simply be too much. As I said earlier, *almost* no one got PTSD from watching TV. It seems the malady requires not only the physiological fear reaction but also the psychological reality of the threat.

A new problem may occur when a person is not able to judge what is real. Mr. Wordsworth was the extreme example of this, but the phenomenon more commonly has been observed in children. A study published by a team of Harvard researchers in 2007 estimated that up to 5 percent of children who repeatedly watched the 9/11 attacks ended up with symptoms similar to PTSD.

"Mr. Addler is asking for Valium," Nurse Season piped in again. "What do we do about that?"

Mr. Addler was not the typical client of the psychiatric hospital. Most of our patients were hospitalized for a relatively brief time, given a helping hand until they could make it back out into their regular lives. There is, after all, nothing magical about hospitalization. We use the same medications, the same therapies, and the same encouragements that a person might receive in an outpatient clinic. The only difference is closer monitoring and a controlled environment. Thus, as soon as they can safely do so, most patients choose to go home. Mr. Addler, however, seemed to like staying with us. He was one of those individuals who, in the old days, probably would have been diagnosed with "nerves." We said he had generalized anxiety disorder and panic attacks. He lived alone, tended to take very poor care of himself, and, even before 9/11, was afraid of almost everything. In short, he was set up to develop post traumatic stress.

"I'm not sure," I answered honestly. "Try and talk him down for a while. I'm going to read up on it."

I felt bad leaving Mr. Addler in distress. On the one hand, it made sense to give him something. Wasn't that what kindly doctors always did in old movies? "I'm going to give this poor woman a sedative" seemed a particularly common reaction to grief or stress in 1950s TV dramas. However, those black-and-white images of the doctor were also interspersed with ads on how good smoking was for you, so perhaps skepticism was in order. I took a deep breath. The first rule of medicine is always "do no harm." Given that I knew that people who drink in the face of disaster do worse, and that Valium and comparable drugs work similar to alcohol, I wasn't sure I would be doing Mr. Addler a favor by giving him what he was asking for.

It turns out there isn't a whole lot of formal research into drugs to prevent PTSD. It is hard to set up scientific review committees amid a catastrophe. The one formal study that looked at benzodiazepines—the class of medications that includes Valium, Xanax, and Klonopin—showed that they had no benefit in preventing post traumatic stress. There were many anecdotal reports of patients liking these medications, of their saying that tranquilizers were the one thing that took the edge off symptoms. Unfortunately, there were at least as many stories of individuals becoming addicted or finding that numbing the symptoms in the short term only prolonged recovery. All in all, it was a very mixed bag.

In reading up on benzodiazepines, I ran across a few other medications that, while still experimental, seem to help without the addictive potential of Valium or its kin.

A type of blood pressure pill called beta-blockers has shown promise. These medications are normally used to slow down the pulse by preventing the effects of adrenaline on the heart, but they also block the effects of noradrenaline, adrenaline's chemical cousin in the brain. Individuals given beta-blockers in emergency rooms immediately after a traumatizing event were found to have lower rates of PTSD than those who got sugar pills.

Similarly, although somewhat counterintuitively, burn victims who were given small amounts of the stress hormone cortisol in the immediate recovery period were found to have reduced rates of PTSD. The reasoning behind this approach is complicated—surges of the hormone during stress suppress both resting levels of the hormone as well as other stress hormones—but it did seem to be a method that worked without risk of addiction.

There is speculation about medications called selective serotonin reuptake inhibitors, or SSRIs. Prozac, Paxil, and Zoloft all fall into this class and have proven, although modest, benefits in established PTSD. Contrary to what Tom Cruise and Scientologists may espouse, they are pretty safe medications and don't have addictive potential. Unfortunately, they have rarely been tested as preventatives for the condition. Any assumptions about whether they would have helped our patients that day are purely conjecture.

I called back Nurse Season to ask. "How's Mr. Addler's blood pressure?"

She took a moment to obtain a check of vital signs. "Through the roof: 160 over 100 with a resting pulse of 110."

"Why don't we treat that first," I suggested. "The beta-blocker might help calm him down at the same time."

An hour later, Mr. Addler's blood pressure and his requests for Valium were both dramatically decreased. Whenever one individual is treated, you can never know whether the response is because of the pill or some other factor. Nurse Season certainly had a calming effect, and, medication-wise, it is possible that if we had given him a Tic-Tac the same effect would have been seen. Placebos are wonderful drugs for anxiety. I do know that, in the end, Mr. Addler didn't end up with PTSD—one bright point in an otherwise awful day.

The day seemed to go on forever. By the end of it, I wasn't much in the mood to celebrate my birthday. A couple of close friends took me out to dinner, but I decided to heed my own advice and stay away from alcohol. Normally, I have nothing against a good party, but in the context of a huge stress, even controlled drinking can lead to trouble. I called it an early night, and September 12 came quickly.

In the morning, I was still shocked and grieving, but the routine went much as it had the day before: alarm, cold floor, shower, dress, listen to the news on the way to work, chat with colleagues while waiting for the morning meeting to begin. People were reacting in different ways. Some wanted to talk. Some were silent. Many prayed for peace and recovery, but being in the military, there was also a clear sense that we were going to have a job to do. A political cartoon that had run in the *San Diego Tribune* gained rapid popularity at the hospital and at other military installations in the area. It was of an eagle sharpening its claws. Prudence dictated that America be sure of its enemy before retaliating, but we were angry. There was no doubt that, one way or another, we were going to war.

Elisabeth Kübler-Ross outlines five stages that people go through in reaction to catastrophic news: denial, followed by anger, followed by bargaining, then depression, and finally acceptance. I seemed to feel these things all at once. There was anger in the actions of wanting to go to war but also acceptance. Risks had to be taken, preparations made. There were a few individuals who could do nothing but curl up and cry, and others who ranted that we should nuke the entire Middle East into a sea of glass. However, most individuals at the hospital, whether patients or staff, simply faced up to the complications of emotions and life. They coped.

In the days, weeks, and months after 9/11, most of us got on with our lives, but we also realized that there were going to be new stresses. Afghanistan had broken the Soviet Army and the British before that. If the United States were to avoid falling victim to the same course of history, we would have to be in top condition. There was a rumor afoot that things were going to get thornier. Whether by inside knowledge or a lucky guess, a guest lecturer in combat medicine ended his talk with a prescient statement.

"You need to be ready to keep treating problems as they arise. It's an open secret that after Afghanistan, we're going into Iraq."

I didn't believe him at the time, but he would be proven right. We would not have just a day of trauma on 9/11 but years of strife. If we were going to avoid creating more Johns and Marias, lifelong PTSD sufferers, we had to know when to start treating. The *Diagnostic and Statistical Manual of Mental Disorders* is somewhat arbitrary in dictating that we call things PTSD if the symptoms have lasted for more than a month, but you do have to draw a line somewhere. We do know that if problems go on as long as three months, PTSD symptoms probably aren't going to remit spontaneously. If this happens, see a doctor.

The single most important thing that I learned from 9/11, however, was that people didn't always need me. They are resilient. There are lots

of different ways of muddling through, lots of different ways of grieving and moving on. We as psychiatrists may have some general advice:
don't drink alcohol, stay in touch with people, keep working, talk to
your doctor. But mental health is the most inexact of sciences. Different
things work for different people. Even if a pattern of familiar symptoms
appears, if it isn't causing impairment, it isn't a disorder. It isn't PTSD. If
you're OK, it's OK.

# 9

# Iraq in Digital

T H E software still has a few glitches," said Dr. Jim Spira as I took off the headset and returned from virtual Baghdad to the quiet of his San Diego office. Jim was seated at the controls of the virtual reality computer, and, despite the neon-green battle going on behind him on the video screens, he radiated his usual sense of calm. Dr. Spira was known in the department as our samurai psychologist, both for his balding pate and for his tendency to bring the teachings from judo and tai chi into therapy sessions. It was easy to envision him meditating in the midst of such a battle.

The world in which I had been immersed was a virtual reality simulator. I had been wearing a headset that looked like sunglasses on steroids. Through these glasses, images of Iraq were projected in front of my eyes. The images were not photorealistic but graphical representations, similar to what you might see in a high-end video game. What made it virtual reality, as opposed to a regular video game, was the way I could interact with the environment. The headset contained a motion sensor. When I turned my head, the computer responded, moving the images to match my movements. From inside the headset, it appeared as if I were interacting with a real, albeit digitally rendered, world.

Headphones produced sound in a similarly three-dimensional manner. The fire to my right would be heard mostly in my right ear, unless
I turned around, in which case the sound would reverse and come in
from the left. As I approached, the sound grew louder. Retreat and both
the sound and vision of the fire would fade into the distance. I had to
use a joystick to "walk" or "drive," since this simulator didn't contain
a treadmill. Instead, I had been standing on what amounted to a giant
subwoofer. It created the rumble of the car's engine and the vibratory
shockwave of the explosive blast. The experience could also be enhanced
by bringing in smells or by changing the lighting or temperature of the
room.

I shrugged. "I'm sure you can fix the bugs, but I still don't understand
how this is going to help someone who's been in combat get over post
traumatic stress disorder."

"It can seem counterintuitive," Dr. Spira conceded. "But we have
been using the virtual reality for years to treat Vietnam Vets and other
trauma survivors. We teach people to confront the things that they are
afraid of. PTSD symptoms build up because you associate real danger
with the type of stimuli you just experienced. If you run through the
same video sequence enough times without that link to real danger, you
realize that the sights and sounds don't hurt you, and it becomes less
scary."

"So if we know it works, why is it research?"

I asked this not merely as a rhetorical question. My job at Naval
Medical Center San Diego was to build a science program. During our
last training review, we had received very high marks for our clinical
work but had been dinged for not doing enough academic research. The
chairman of Psychiatry had offered me a job based on the proposition
that I build a mental health research team at the hospital. Luckily, it
turned out, two other people in the department were already way ahead
of me on this idea.

Jim Spira was one of these pioneers. The other was Jeff Pyne, an
always-smiling man who sat behind Jim as the VR system was demonstrated. Jeff was a Navy reservist who had been called up to work at
Naval Medical Center San Diego. In his regular civilian life, Dr. Pyne
was a full-time researcher at the Department of Veterans Affairs Hospital

in Arkansas. He had a list of grants and publications that outshone just about anyone in the Navy. He had been offered the research director job before I was but had turned it down in favor of returning to Arkansas with his bride. His imminent departure didn't stop him from getting things ready for his replacement. He had called up the Office of Naval Research (ONR) and asked them what they would be interested in funding.

"It turns out virtual reality is a hot topic," Dr. Pyne explained. "It's like a solution in search of a problem. ONR is interested in advancing the technology for a number of reasons, and the new director there, Commander Shilling, is a psychologist. He knows about all the existing work with VR and PTSD and wants to push the envelope. Technically, we are funded for software development, but we get to do good science in the process."

"So most of the money would go to the companies that build the VR systems?"

"A fair amount of it, but they were the ones who did the work in putting together the original proposals anyway. It really is a win–win for you. They do the paperwork. Jim runs the day-to-day management of the program. The department gets new therapists paid for by the grant, and you get enough seed money to start your new research section."

I was still skeptical. I had envisioned a program that compared the existing treatments for PTSD. With a flood of patients coming in, I thought the question that needed to be answered was what should we use now, not what can we develop that might work years down the line. I had to admit that the VR program sounded like a good deal, but there is an expression about things that seem too good to be true.

"So what do you need me for?" I asked.

Jim looked sheepish. "Well, politics," he said. "You know I don't get along so well with our illustrious leader."

"Politics and media," Jeff added. "They want someone in uniform to be in the pictures, and I'll be gone by the time the project comes through."

"Media? You won't get any real data on this project for at least two years. We don't have any results to show them," I scoffed. I had been involved in exciting findings before, but it was always like pulling teeth to get the press interested in science. And that was when we had real findings to show.

A series of animated explosions flashed on the multiple video screens set up in the lab. "They are already coming to us," Jim smiled the sheepish grin again. "Reporters love cool toys."

"That, and the software developers have talent for press," Jeff added. "One of the scientists down at the University of Southern California is a technology reporter's fantasy. Name is Skip Rizzo. He rides a Harley, dresses like a rock star, and his lab looks like it's from the *Starship Enterprise*. The press has been all over him. He wants to show off the stuff he is building here for the military."

"I thought you said the software developers were named, what was it, Wiederhold?"

"That's the other company," Jeff explained. "There are two groups that put in grants and want us to test their systems. Brenda and Mark Wiederhold are two doctors here in San Diego who own a company called Virtual Reality Medical Center. Dr. Rizzo is under contract to another company called Virtually Better from Atlanta. The two companies normally hate each other, but they have cooperated to put together this prototype for us."

"Our collaborators hate each other, and I'm going to be the one who is supposed to handle the politics?" I said, realizing that all my sentences lately had been ending in question marks. "What are they feuding about?"

"Not really sure," said Jeff. "They're all nice and very intelligent people, and on the face of it, they seem to agree on ninety-nine percent of everything about VR."

My wariness was starting to get stronger. "And the other one percent?"

"It's largely a question of direction. The Wiederholds have been working with Virtual Reality for years. They started off using it to treat phobias, fear of flying and such. They would teach people to relax using biofeedback, and then introduce them to the virtual reality environment as a place to practice their skills before they had to get aboard an actual airplane. They have taken this concept and applied it to PTSD. The Virtually Better team, on the other hand, has Barbara Rothbaum as its guru. She is a PTSD expert and was part of the first group to apply VR to PTSD.

In her method, VR is added to what was already known to be one of the best therapies for the condition, prolonged exposure therapy. She has the patients tell their trauma stories over and over out loud while they are in the simulation. Habituation kicks in eventually, and the fear diminishes."

"Habituation, like for sound?" I continued my run of uninterrupted interrogatives.

Habituation was something they taught about in introductory psychology classes to explain aspects of attention. Anyone who has been around a construction site will recognize the phenomenon. If there is a series of loud sounds, for example, explosions, separated by random periods of time, a person will start to become more and more focused on them. He will wait for the next bang. On the other hand, if the sounds are continuous—for example, like the sound of a jackhammer—the brain will start to accept the sound as part of the background, and, soon, you won't even hear it anymore.

"It turns out habituation works for fear as well," Jeff explained. "If you are around something long enough and nothing bad happens, your brain gets used to it. Think about it. There is basically no fear of heights in cliff-dwelling communities. It is something they are used to. In Western society, consider our relationship with roads. Standing next to a freeway is just as dangerous as standing at a cliff's edge. But since we do it all the time, it doesn't bother us."

I nodded. This fit well with what I already knew about the cycle of avoidance in PTSD. The more a person tries not to think about the trauma, the stronger the memory seems to get. It is as if the brain learns to classify what is dangerous based on what we avoid. Running away from thoughts inside our own heads doesn't work well. It only reenforces the idea that the thought is to be feared and leaves the sufferer waiting for the next explosion of memory.

"The two virtual reality methods seem pretty similar," I said. "I guess it's true what they say about academics. The feuds are so big because the stakes are so small."

Jeff laughed. "I think the feud goes beyond the science, but in both methods, the use of the VR machine means that you can control the environment so the patients can't avoid their fears. You can push them until they have to apply the skill or ability to relax and habituate."

"We prefer to think of it as the patient pushing himself," Jim corrected. "It is ultimately in his or her control. One of the great things about VR is that the patient can let us know if the machine needs to be shut off."

"Well, part of being a scientist is that I'm always willing to give new ideas a shot," I said. "When do you think we will have outcome data so we can evaluate if this is actually a good idea?"

Again the sheepish look. "We're only in the clinical stage at this point," Jim explained. "We don't have IRB approval yet."

I sighed. IRB stands for institutional review board. I sometimes called it our research prevention department. It is ironic that, if an individual doctor wants to try out a therapy or medication with a patient, he may do so as long as the two understand and agree what is going on. This takes about ten minutes. If, on the other hand, the doctor wants to formally test whether the treatment is working, it requires volumes of paperwork, hours of extra training and review, and approval by a collection of individuals that seems specifically composed so that they will never agree on anything. This process can take months or sometimes years.

Science has had its share of excesses and moral outrages, so I wasn't questioning the need to have IRB approval. It is a necessary evil. Frustrated researchers often note, however, that the original tests for penicillin or the smallpox vaccine would never have made it past a modern review board. As for psychology experiments, well, the more ethically controversial of those seemed to have migrated out of the laboratory and onto reality TV. I hoped that we weren't playing into that trend by getting ourselves involved with the media so early.

"So we are going to the press with absolutely no results to talk about?"

Again the fireworks on the video screen. "We do have something to show," Jim said. "And I have had clinical success with the treatment."

Jeff's smile was still there despite my obvious ongoing discomfort. He knew I was hooked. "Better break out your dress blues," he said.

I sent my dress uniform to the dry cleaners. I tried to bone up on the background as best I could while we waited for the interviews to be arranged and the IRB approval to come through. I was still interested in trying to get drug trials off the ground, but the more I read, the more I realized that therapy tended to have better success rates in PTSD than did the medications. I sat in on a few sessions of therapy Jim was conducting and arranged to learn the other technique from Dr. Rothbaum and another collaborator at Cornell University, JoAnn Difede, who had been using VR therapy with survivors of the attacks on the World Trade Center. That team had impressive results. They made a strong argument for why existing techniques to treat PTSD were good but why VR might be better.

In the traditional method of exposure therapy, patients are asked to imagine their traumas long enough for habituation to kick in. They are also asked to go out and find real-world situations that remind them of their traumas and face up to them. What if a patient is unable or unwilling to maintain the imagined image? What if facing the real situation would put the individual's life at risk again? Virtual reality could solve both these problems. The image would be maintained as long as the computer was on. In the virtual world, even the most dangerous battlefield could be challenged without risk of harm.

In *The Matrix*, individuals who die in a computer simulation die in real life. That was clearly untrue of our virtual reality simulations. It did seem, however, that the experience could be overwhelming for some individuals. The very name *virtual reality* challenges philosophical ideas about what *real* means. In general, experiences perceived through sensory input and which are reported in the same way by different individuals are called *real*. If one person sees and feels a tree, but others do not, we call it a hallucination. If everyone sees and feels that tree, we call that tree *real*. In VR, individuals can share the same sensory experience of something we all objectively know is a simulation.

As the project progressed, the simulations became more and more real. The two companies split off in different directions in terms of what their software would reproduce. The team from Virtually Better focused on creating combat scenarios for Soldiers and Marines. These were detailed, including not only the sights and sounds of combat but also a smell machine and a large vibrating platform, which could re-create the rumble of a tactical vehicle or the shock wave of a distant explosion. The team from Virtual Reality Medical Center had been charged with creating simulations for support staff, the engineers, medics, mechanics, translators, and others who were less likely to be involved in direct combat but who might suffer trauma in diverse ways. They had to build more scenarios and did not have time for smell or the rumble of the earth. A virtual hospital was built complete with screaming patients. A marketplace offered hidden danger along with Middle Eastern spices. Iraqi homes or a base camp—each place was designed to trigger and help control the weight of memory.

As the technology became more exciting, reporters became more interested. CBS, NBC, ABC, Fox, NPR, the *Washington Post, Salon* magazine, even MTV and *GQ* requested interviews. Everyone wanted to try on the goggles and get shot at—everyone, that is, except those who had actually been to war. Most reporters enjoyed the experience. An exception, and this would actually come much later, was when Sanjay Gupta of CNN tried out the simulation. Dr. Gupta had been a correspondent in Iraq and had famously performed surgery in the field when it turned out he was the only neurosurgeon available in an isolated section of that country. In his blog, Gupta would later describe his experience trying out the VR:

> I wasn't ready for what would happen to my mind and body. Through this technology, which is like a video game and experienced by the patient wearing a wired-up helmet, I truly relived some of the most terrifying moments of my life, those moments when I really thought I was going to die.

It turns out that virtual reality is much more realistic for someone who has been sensitized to the experience. In early work with VR, our collaborators had discovered an interesting phenomenon. In an attempt to treat fear of flying, they had run individuals through a simulation of an airplane flight. This used much more primitive technology than we now had available. A very blocky, blurry flight attendant came down the aisle as the virtual flight progressed. The software was not sophisticated enough for her to actually offer drinks or to interact with the passengers. It was definitely not to the point where a smell machine had been built in. However, those patients with a flying phobia reported that they actually smelled coffee as the flight attendant passed. They saw not what was in the virtual simulation but the fears that plagued their own minds.

This was greatly exaggerated when we stepped up from treating phobias to treating PTSD. This didn't change the fact that the treatment was effective. Those in the airplane simulation overcame their fear of flying. Dr. Gupta, too, was able to rapidly adapt to the VR world:

> I could feel my heart pound and my hands shake as the therapist continued to remind me that the purpose of the simulation is to let me experience those moments as realistically as possible, but in a safe place. I was overwhelmed by my response to this experimental treatment. I felt so out of control with real feelings of helplessness and despair at first. I felt more in control after going through the simulation a couple more times.

I never clinically interviewed Dr. Gupta, but given that he showed no signs of impairment in his life, it was doubtful that he was actually suffering from full-blown PTSD. If it was that scary for him, how much harder would it be to enter this virtual world for someone who had been debilitated by his or her trauma?

The lack of IRB approval for the project was becoming more of a frustration. As the press mounted and the data lagged, tempers frayed. Was the therapy actually effective in our patients? We needed to know.

"I'm quitting," Jim said as I came into his office as we prepared for another interview.

"Very funny," I said. "I talked to the Clinical Investigation Department today. They said that our IRB approval should come through any day now. We've lined up some good therapists to start working on the VR with you. I'm hoping by next month, when you are up and running, I'll finally be able to start on my other projects. This virtual reality stuff has eaten our lives, hasn't it?"

"No. I'm serious. I'm quitting. I lined up another job. It's a great opportunity, and they're going to let me write my own work schedule."

I'm not sure of the number of times we went back and forth before I realized that he really was serious.

"I won't abandon you on this," he said. "We can call and talk about the projects anytime you want, but I'm afraid you are going to have to run them."

"But, Jim, I haven't treated a single person with the VR. How am I supposed to run the project without you here?"

He radiated that calm of his again. "I guess you'll learn."

# IO

# Women at War

SORRY again, Ma'am." David nodded to the tall, red-headed woman next to him. He had just used an expletive to describe Ramadi, a city in Iraq.

"You don't have to apologize to me," Ruby responded. "I was there too, and that's about the way I would put it. And you don't need to call me 'Ma'am.' I'm enlisted."

"Yeah," David looked at the ground, appearing embarrassed. "Sorry about that too. Most of the women I've known in the military have been nurses, officers."

There was an awkward silence.

David and Ruby were part of our combat PTSD group. A couple of years had passed since I first observed Dr. Slier organize this type of activity, and I was now running one of my own. People came in civilian clothes and went by their first names. Anonymity prevented difficulties when a private was talking to a major, but it also meant it was harder to read backgrounds. Slacks and a t-shirt don't come with medals or a combat infantry badge.

"Ruby," I said. "You've been a trailblazer in the group. You were the first woman here. Was that hard for you?"

"No, she wasn't the first," interrupted another of the group's members from the other side of the circle. "There was that other girl, I mean woman, back when Dr. Oliver was running the group."

"That one was a nurse, I think," said a fourth voice.

"Not a nurse, a corpsman."

"I thought she was a Seabee, but she only came the one time. Must not have liked us."

"She did say we were part of the problem. She called Bill an a—hole. Again, sorry about the language, Ruby."

I raised my hand to cut off the banter from the male participants. "Ruby, you didn't answer the question. Is it hard being the only woman in the group?"

Ruby shot daggers in my direction but then answered with a shrug. "Naw. I like you a—holes."

Laughter went round the circle, diffusing the tension.

"Yeah," said Bill, slapping Ruby on the back. "Ruby is just another one of the guys."

For a moment, Ruby turned as red as her hair. Whether this was from embarrassment at the comment or anger at the slap (most people with PTSD don't like to be touched suddenly), I wasn't sure. Either way, she rapidly recovered and joined in the round of friendly insults. "One of the a—holes you mean, one of the a—holes from f—king Ramadi."

The group laughed again, and the conversation turned back to the serious topic of why particular cities in Iraq had been more miserable than others. Ruby's swearing had seemed to me an attempt to fit in, to be "one of the guys," but I chose not to challenge it for now. Discussion or process groups such as this weren't really considered an essential place for treatment change to occur. Rather, they were set up so that Service Members with PTSD could feel supported by their comrades in arms. I knew that it was harder for Ruby, but I also knew that she didn't want to be different. But things for women in the military have always been a little different.

During the Revolutionary War, George Washington authorized women to be attached to the Continental Army but only as nurses, cooks, laundresses, and water bearers. Officially, these were all "support roles" and were meant to keep women out of the line of fire. Even then, war didn't always shoot so straight. In 1776, Margaret Corbin became the first woman to be officially wounded in US combat. She had been stationed with her husband at Fort Tryon, New York. The fort was assaulted, and Margaret's husband was killed while manning a cannon. Margaret, seeing him fall, took up the position at the cannon against the Hessian invaders and continued firing until she herself was wounded. She was captured by the British Army, held as a prisoner of war, and eventually released. In 1779, Congress awarded her a pension. There is now a famous statue of her at West Point, although it wasn't until 1968 that the Military Service Academy started admitting women for officer training.

Today, women serve as fighter pilots, military police, commanding officers, and many other rolls. Sixteen percent of the military is female. The Coast Guard has no gender-restricted jobs, and the Air Force opens 99 percent of its positions to women. Previously all-male bastions, such as submarine service, are rapidly opening to gender equality. Only frontline ground jobs such as the infantry, tank units, Special Forces, and combat engineers are still restricted to men. Even for those positions, women sometimes fill in, since in a war with no front line, what is the difference between "frontline combat" and "rear area security"? Still, Ruby's position in feeling apart was not unusual for women in combat. "Female boots on enemy ground" was a concept that the military was still getting used to.

"I know that y'all were there," one group member tried to apologize to Ruby. "It was just that we never saw women. Not during the invasion at least, or not unless we were wounded."

It was not unusual for men in the initial invasions of Iraq or Afghanistan to go through their entire deployment without having contact with a female Service Member. The exception in these wars, as in many before it, was for medical providers. Caregivers were in too short a supply to let ideas about gender get in the way of saving lives. In the Vietnam War, all the female Service Members killed in combat were nurses. There are still many women in military medicine. There have to be. Half of all medical school graduates are women. More than 70 percent of psychologists are female, and in nursing, women outnumber men fifteen to one.

Many of my female colleagues were part of the initial invasions of

Iraq and Afghanistan. At the mental health clinic in Fallujah where I served in 2008, the psychologist was Dr. Colleen Barnum. This five-foot-tall spitfire of a woman often went out on daily convoys to be with the troops while I was more safely entrenched in camp. She often went on these trips in the required fire-resistant suit, which until about half-way through the deployment was a one-piece outfit. It hadn't occurred to anyone that for a woman to go to the bathroom would require taking the entire thing off. Although serious oversights like this were still present, what had changed by 2008 was that the medical providers weren't the only women in camp. Our guards, construction workers, communications officers, and even pilots were often women. As of June 2010, 113 women had been killed in Iraq and Afghanistan, and they came from all walks of life.

After that day's session, I started thinking about the other female member of the group, the one who had left. They said she was a Seabee. Construction battalion is abbreviated "CB," and the term was so commonly mistaken to be an ocean insect that the units eventually gave in to the nomenclature. Seabees were always part of the war but became particularly important when efforts shifted from invasion to reconstruction and fortification. As "noncombat" units, they are gender-integrated. Unfortunately, stationary reconstruction projects are enticing targets for hit-and-run raids, and the convoys on which they travel are frequently hit by improvised explosive devices or other attacks. A female Seabee was one of the first PTSD patients that we treated with virtual reality. She had been hit by IEDs at least five times on deployments. I didn't think it was her, but the comments in the group made me think of a different Service Member who had come through our clinic. I wondered if it might not be coincidence.

"Lois," I asked at our next appointment. "You mentioned before that you had tried the PTSD groups, but didn't like them. Can you tell me about that?"

"Yeah," Lois settled her muscular frame into the chair across from me. She had been a construction worker even before joining the Navy, and before she was injured in Afghanistan had prided herself on being able to outlift most men on a job. "Groups aren't my thing. My situation's too, shall we say, complex for them."

"You mean in that that you are both a combat Veteran and a sexual assault survivor?"

Lois was dealing with what is sometimes called complex PTSD, that is, post traumatic stress that stems from more than one source of trauma. It is possible that complex PTSD is the rule, not the exception, since there appears to be a cumulative effect of trauma in creating the disorder. Although exact statistics are disputed, childhood trauma appears more common in girls, and, as adults, women are more likely to be the victims of sexual assault. According to a report by the Family Violence Prevention Fund, annual sexual assault rates are 2 for every 1,000 female Service Members, versus 1.8 per 1,000 civilian women and 1 per 1,000 civilian men.

"That's part of it," Lois said. "I never felt I fit in to either the combat groups or the women's groups, and I was already sick of trying so hard to fit in. The military and construction are both mostly made up of men. As a woman, there are a few ways you can adapt. You can ignore it and try to be you. That works fine as long as you can carry all the weight yourself. You can become one of the guys. I did that by naturally being so big and by being a weightlifter. People sometimes assumed I was a lesbian. Strange as it may sound, it might have made it easier if I was. The guys at a construction site would have loved it if I had joined them in making catcalls. The construction workers, the guys in the combat groups, they wanted to make me into one of them, only with breasts. The thing is, I am a woman, and I want to stay that way."

I wasn't sure I agreed with Lois about it being easier if she had been a lesbian. I had several homosexual patients who struggled with being part of an institution that made them hide their sexuality and spouses. For now, however, I was more interested in how Lois was struggling to find her identity.

"And the women's groups? You didn't feel they were supportive either?"

"They tried to be, I suppose, but in the end they pissed me off too. I mean, I say I want to be thought of as a woman, but I'm not into the 'rah-rah sisterhood' thing either. I can't stand the way some women's organizations assume the military is all bad. Hell, let's be honest, half the military is teenagers, and there is going to be some voluntary sex going

on. When there are fifty guys to every gal on deployment, some women
do get hooked on all the attention, and start sleeping with everything
that moves. The military regs against fraternization and adultery are
there for a reason. I followed those regs. I felt like what happened to me
was partly the fault of the way a few of these women acted."

"So you feel that both groups tried to make you ally against a part of
yourself?"

"More that they both included people who seemed like the ones responsible for what happened to me. I want to be both a Sailor and a
woman, and I found that when I was around them, I was hating both."

"But surely some part of you was also proud of both?"

"Oh, sure," Lois nodded. "I'm sure I don't need to tell you about all
the brave things that I saw Sailors and Soldiers do. They give medals for
that. Maybe they should give an award for holding up as a lady in the
military, the pink heart they could call it, or the stone skin if the other's
too girly for you. I mean, it takes a pretty thick skin to put up with the
harassment, and the belittling, and the crap you take as a woman in any
workplace, but then to go out and almost get killed defending the Saudi
or the Kuwait border only to be told that when you are in that country
there, you aren't allowed to drive."

"So that's the stone skin," I said. "What about the pink heart?"

Lois paused for a moment, a long moment. I wasn't sure she was going
to go on. Did she think I was making fun of her? No, she looked very
serious in her response.

"It's hard to keep your heart," she said. "I saw women who did things
in Afghanistan, no man could have done. When we went into the
schools, I know we were an inspiration to those girls. We were just as
tough, and we showed them that America could care. I saw women keep
each other sane. When there are so few of you, you have to lean on each
other, and sometimes military rules about fraternization among ranks
make that risky. If there are only two women in a unit, and one's a major
and one's a private, you aren't supposed to be friends, but women found
ways of supporting each other anyway. I know that there were times that
walking to the showers with another gal kept me from getting harassed
by the guys, and hell, maybe I would have been raped even earlier if it
hadn't been for that kind of protection in numbers. Before all this, I did

have a heart. I trusted that the military was made up of gentleman and ladies. But it's made up of people.

"I had this idea, thought that women were better. But, the thing about war is that we are killing people too. We are doing all the brave things the men are, but the terrible things too. Remember that picture that made the news of the female private who had those Iraqi prisoners on a leash? That isn't half of it. We go out and are Mother America in the Arabic schools, and then we go back and load the shells that land on those kids' homes the next night. What is that they always say in those rape prevention ads? It could be your mother, your sister, your daughter, right? How many people have their mother, sister, or daughter blowing the head off an Afghan kid when he tries to sneak in over the wire one night?"

"Was that you? Did you blame yourself for having to do a job that potentially involved killing? You know it wasn't your fault, right?"

"Yeah, I know that. But I'm not even a killer. I never had to fire my weapon. I did build schools, but in the military, you are either a killer or a pussy, and that's what they saw me as, pussy, a target, not one them of them at all. And it wasn't only the man who raped me. It was all the people who stood by, the men and the women, the people who could have done something. The war showed me that anyone can be a monster, them, us, men, women, hell, even the kids. The boy who jumped the fence was strapped with explosives. I had this idea of myself as strong and good. But I see what I see, and I have to ask myself, which is it? Am I weak? Am I evil? Why are the Afghanis trying to kill me, and my own shipmates raping me? I feel like I was a naïve little girl, and I ask, can I ever be that lady I once thought I could be?"

"And yet you haven't left," I pointed out. "You were promoted a month or so ago, as I remember?"

"Yeah," Lois nodded, almost smiled. "Moving up the ranks," she said. "If things are ever going to change, we women are going to have to stick around. We are going to have to remind the men that the military isn't a frat party with guns. We matter, and we have good ideas. The very idea of being an officer and a gentleman came about when someone thought that knights might be put to better use defending women rather than attacking them. Now the guys are going to have to get used to the idea that we are knights, too, that we are defending each other. Maybe we can find a way of being fierce and protective all at the same time."

"That's a pretty good speech," I said. "Do you think you might give it at group some time?"

"Maybe," she said. "I've got a plan to change the military and the world. You want me to fix myself, too?"

"I do," I said.

And then there were two women in our PTSD group.

# I I

# Memorial Day in Camp Fallujah

IT is hard to avoid death in a war zone. Monuments and plaques indicated places where comrades had fallen in camp. Pockmarked walls and hospital statistics marked the sheer volume of carnage that had happened here. Everyone knows someone who has died. Most days you put it behind you. But certain days are set aside. These are days for grief.

On Memorial Day 2008, thousands of Service Members filed into the Chapel of Hope in Camp Fallujah, an amphitheater captured during the invasion and converted to that purpose. No one was required to come, but almost every man and woman who was not on duty attended the memorial. There are rules written and unwritten in the military and some that are just known. The seats of the chapel were filled with Soldiers, Sailors, Airmen, and Marines, different shades of camouflage. Most Service Members had put on a pressed uniform, but others had come recently from the field, their faces and clothing still covered with the dust, smoke, and oil of the Iraqi desert. The service started, and it was, sadly, familiar to all.

The ceremony for the Memorial Day service was the same as for individual funerals in theater. Everyone stood at attention. A hymn was sung. At the front of the room, the implements of the dead Service Member were brought forth—a rifle, a helmet, boots, dog tags. The rifle was placed bayonet down in the earth, the other pieces positioned in their proper places on and around the weapon. The symbols of the Warrior were saluted.

As the symbolic grave stood at the front of the chapel, images of the dead Service Members were shown. Those still bearing arms looked on the faces of the fallen while the chaplain gave a sermon. He talked about the dead and the living, and the commanding officer spoke about the purpose for which these young men and women died. Roll call was sounded. The names at the end gave no answer. A bugle called the slow lament.

Grief doesn't always fall within the realm of mental health. Unlike PTSD or major depressive disorder, conditions that imply an impairment that must be overcome, grief is not always something from which a person wants to recover. Grief can be a memorial, as much a reminder as the rifle and empty boots, that there once was a vital person on this earth who should not have left it so early.

There is no cure for grief, no pill or therapy session that makes it OK that young men and women die. There are parts to grieving that some have found useful—ceremony, memorial, faith, a commitment to live up to the ideals for which the person died. So much has been written and said about grief that I would do it a disservice to try to sum it up in a paragraph or two. I will say that combat adds its own complexities to the grieving process.

There is the scale. How do you mourn for thousands? Beyond this is the connection. The memorial service in Fallujah was held in a combat zone. A single shell could have come in and wiped out the entire service. Many there that day had lived through the same firefights or IED blasts that killed those mourned. Many more were leaving to face the same dangers. The service reminded us all not just of loss but of mortality and the proximity we had to it each day.

Finally, there is the meaning of being a Warrior. These men and women had not been killed by random chance, by old age, or by disease, but by an enemy determined to pursue us to our graves. We would do our best to end them first. If for revenge, or duty, or justice, or a need to protect our own loved ones, we were still sworn to leave the enemy's widows and orphans mourning. How do you find peace when there is still death in your heart?

After the memorial, I went looking for one of the chaplains who ran the service. The senior of these, Captain Pusateri, was kind enough to comply. He was a tall, thin man, with a gray crew cut and a strong voice that carried in church or in his office. He used that voice to welcome me. I asked him if there were things that chaplains knew that we psychiatrists did not. I asked him why we went to such lengths to cultivate and memorialize our pain. I asked him how he could be a man of faith in a place where forgiveness was not currently an option.

The chaplain answered slowly. "There are questions that have no answers. I know. I've asked them myself. When I was in the first Gulf War, I was working closely with a squadron, and every day one of my friends would not come home. I'd question why they died, why I lived. I'm in a different position now, but the questions are still the same. How could this have happened? How can I possibly get over this?

"During my last deployment in Iraq, we had a tragic event. All events in war are tragic, but this one stuck out for the bad luck of it all. The Corporal that died, he was a favorite of the unit, really beloved. His platoon was getting ready to go home. They had served a hard tour, and lost a lot of men, but it seemed like the worst was over. They were careful. They were staying inside the wire. Four Marines were up in the guard tower the last night, joking with each other. Sniper fire came in. The shots were from so far away that no one ever knew where they came from. There was no way that someone could have aimed from that distance, but the Corporal, he was hit.

"The young man was struck in the throat. The bullet hit in a spot where the body armor doesn't cover. His death wasn't instant, but he never had a chance. There is too much that can be broken in a man's throat. All of his blood came pouring out, and it sprayed over the other three.

"The three survivors were badly shaken. Not only had they lost a friend, a man with whom, moments before, they were sharing stories about what they would do when they got home; they all knew that it could have been any of them. A step to the left, or a gust of wind that changed the drift of the bullet, and there would have been a different outcome. Maybe all of them would have lived. Maybe the blood covering the guard shack, and the tears that came from the survivors, they would have come from different men.

"I was asked to come in to try and help them. Each of the three found solace in a different way. I met with the trio, and then we talked individually over the next few days. They each had been in the same place, only a few feet from each other, but it is amazing how differently they saw the situation.

"The senior man in the group was a Staff Sergeant. He'd been deployed before and had seen other men killed. He was the most directly appreciative of my visit.

" 'So God has come into the room,' he said when I arrived.

"I know that he was joking with me, but I also know that he was being somewhat serious. A chaplain is a visible reminder of values. It's an odd sort of symbolism when you think about it. We chaplains are all men of faith, but often very different faiths. At that point, he didn't know if I was Catholic or Protestant. Unless he looked closely at my insignia, he probably didn't even know if I was a priest, a rabbi, or an imam. Even for the atheist, we represent hope that maybe there is a greater plan in it all, that fragile flesh and blood is not all there is.

"Death, horror, it shakes our sense of how the universe is supposed to work. It is so wrong. The Staff Sergeant felt this. There were tears pouring down his face, but he was able to still love God even when He had hurt him. This is the lesson of Job. Job, like the wise Staff Sergeant, never would curse God. For all His works that seemed unexplainable, He offered purpose, a way to get at that unanswerable question. I didn't tell the Staff Sergeant that it was all part of God's plan. I've seen other chaplains do this, and personally I think it is a mistake. People resist meaning if you try to thrust it on them. I prefer to listen, because I carry all the message I need to when I reach out for their hand. If they are ready for it, they will hear that small, still voice that whispers God's meaning. I don't have to say a thing.

"For the second man, faith wasn't so easy. He was angry. This was a young man, a Lance Corporal, slightly junior to the one who had died. I had never seen him come to church, and the only time God came up in his language was if it was attached to a 'damn.'

" 'I want to kill them all,' he said. 'I want to tear out their eyes. I want to kill every man, woman, and child in this godforsaken country.'

"Whereas the Staff Sergeant had described every detail in the face of the Corporal who died, the Lance Corporal was focused outward. It infuriated him that he could not tell where the shot came from. He went over this again and again, looking at the way the blood had spattered and which way the wind was blowing, even weighing the quality of the darkness that night and how this would have influenced a sniper's choice of position.

"'Someone smarter than me will figure it out,' he said finally. 'We'll do it right. Just retribution. No better friend. No worse enemy.'

"*Semper fidelis.* I answered the one Marine Corps motto with another. It means always faithful. Being a Marine does not mean being religious, but it does imply a certain level of belief. There is a code, a faith in something larger than yourself, a belief in what is right. I wonder if this is the reason the word *Marine* is always capitalized. For the few and the proud, faith in the corps can be like His word. As a chaplain, I hope that God always comes first, but as a man who served with the Marines, I can understand how it was the corps that held the Lance Corporal together.

"I don't mean to imply that it is only the Marines who can pull this off. I've seen it also in the Army, Air Force, Navy, even in civilians who profess a certain code. There is a code in being an American, a sense that you are connected through history and tradition, through belief, even if that belief has nothing more in common than the sense that we are all entitled to our own faith, or its absence.

"We have developed a number of new ceremonies during the wars in Iraq and Afghanistan. We hold not only the funerals for the families in the States but also a service in the country where the Service Member died. What you saw on Memorial Day is a new tradition, but it always seems old.

"Ceremony connects us to history. Even for the agnostic, these services are important. They remind even the atheist that there is something larger than the self. And it is so important that they are done right. There is a sense that no matter how badly everything else went wrong, that when it comes to burying our dead, we will do things right. We will show honor, and in doing so, we may keep ourselves sane.

"They say that funerals are for the living, not the dead. I think they are for both. We cannot forget our connections to the dead, but also we must remember that it is the living who are still there to hold us up.

"With the third man I met that day, I saw the importance of the connection among comrades. The third survivor was a Corporal, the same rank as the man who died. He had probably been the closest to him of any of the three, but he was the least shaken when I arrived on the scene.

"The surviving Corporal was surrounded by his buddies. They were telling stories about the man who had died, how he was always the first one to volunteer for work, the last one to say a harsh word about anyone. They were also passing around drinks and talking. The drinks weren't alcoholic. We were still in Iraq and liquor was prohibited. This was pure sustenance. There are basic things a human body needs: food, water, sleep, companionship. Here they were getting all these things. There is no way to overemphasize how important they are. You can't live, and you can't heal without them.

"I was a stranger to this group, so I just observed, and when they let me, I shook the men's hands and gave them my condolences.

"'I'm sorry for your loss, Lance Corporal,' I said.

"He answered with a solemn and serene voice. 'Yes, we all are.'

"'We all are.' What powerful words. We find solace and support in each other. We know this, but combat can take that from us. One of the hardest things about war is how removed it seems from the normal course of human events. A Service Member can return home feeling like an alien species, speaking a language and thinking thoughts that no one else can possibly understand. I can't tell you how many times I've heard Service Members say that when they got home, someone asked them about the war, but they felt that the other person didn't really want to know. They have to keep it secret.

"The great thing about comrades in arms is that they already know what you went through. They were there too. The blood that was on that Corporal was also on every man in that circle. They had already seen the body. They knew what the dead man had been like. They were sharing, but at the same time, it was something they already had in common. Each knew the other was still human, and that made it OK to be human too.

"Buddies help in all steps of the process. People who come home together in ships do better than those who fly back alone. People who were dropped newly into a unit do far worse than those who had time to build bonds. When a unit is devastated, there is survivor's guilt. A person can feel like he is the only one left, even when other survivors are reaching out to him. Other times there is a sense of betrayal, an event has made you revile your former friends. Whatever the reason, a person who cuts himself off from the rest of the world pays an awful price. It is a terrible irony that isolation is itself a burden that is too heavy to carry alone.

"There are always opportunities for fellowship. When unit cohesion breaks down, a strong commander can build it up again with a sense of common purpose. A chaplain like me can invite a person to church, not even so much for the service, but for the experience of sitting next to other sinners and souls. Family dinners are wonderful, a chance to be viewed not as a curiosity, but as the person you always were. Even something as simple as a baseball game can do it. One man went to war. The other did not, but they both root for the home team.

"Each of these three men found their way back through a different path. There are probably many others, and I know that sometimes all the faith, or fellowship, or military ethos will not be sufficient. If you listen though, the sufferers may well tell you what they need. If they don't, well, you may have given it to them anyway. The human species has been dealing with death for as long as we have been human. There is something in us that knows what to do and what to feel. Death itself guides us."

As I left the chaplain's office, I remembered my own first experience with death in theater. A badly burned man was rushed through the hospital doors at dusk. Our staff had been extensively trained for the possibility of casualties, but you can never be truly ready. The reduction in hostilities meant that our team had been cut to half of its previous strength. This, in turn, required that every person there had to be trained for the worst. Psychiatrists, psychologists, dentists, even our entomologist learned the basics of putting in an IV and triaging, choosing who has a chance and who needs to be left to die so that more might live.

We all went to our stations, but as it became apparent that there was only one casualty, those of us less skilled at surgery stood back and let the seasoned ER physicians do their work. They bandaged and placed the necessary breathing tubes and other life-stabilizing devices. There was a flurry of activity and then a rush of exaltation as the sounds of a helicopter landing interrupted the chaos. The patient was going to get out alive. For a moment, exaltation overcame the sharp smell of burned flesh and cordite that permeated the building. The patient left the ER still breathing, and young corpsmen felt that they had come through their first test. They had, perhaps, but the patient had not.

There is an image of medicine, perpetuated by television dramas and to a lesser extent by real statistics from injuries stateside, that implies that if you can get a patient to a doctor fast enough, he will live. The fact is that, medicine or no, all of us die. If you are a burn victim, death happens much more quickly and more often. There is a rule of thumb in emergency medicine. Chance of survival is inversely related to the percentage of the body that is burned and to the patient's age.

We didn't know the patient's age at the time or even his name. His ID and dog tags had melted or fallen away in the inferno that consumed him. We did know that he had been charred over most of his body. Only minimal smoke stains had been seen inside his mouth, meaning that he had not been breathing while much of the fire raged. Also, his body was riddled with bullets. These were not from a direct attack. His vehicle had been hit by an unmanned improvised explosive device, but like all good Marines, he had carried a trove of weapons and ammunition with him as he traveled. The fire had cooked these to explosion. Scores of un-aimed rounds fired from their casings and ricocheted inside the armored car. No one lives through that.

By morning, in a hospital room in Baghdad, our patient had joined the ranks of the honored dead. We knew more about him at that point. He was a captain in the Marines. He had a family, children. I searched the news for a story about his death on the Internet. I was sure that it would be there. I could not find a thing. Eventually, I found a webpage called iCasualties that kept track of every one of the fallen. Our captain had been number 4,001.

As I looked over the webpage, and all the other names, a realization struck me. Four thousand dead is, by most estimations of war, pretty good. Fifty-eight thousand US Service Members died in Vietnam, al-most half a million in World War II. Casualty rates were dropping to record lows this year. Still, except for one month, December 2007, every month of the Iraq war had more deaths than days. The major's death was not news because it had become commonplace.

In the abstract, we all know that men die in battle every day. I certainly knew this. But when faced with a man's rifle down in the earth, the smell of his burned flesh still fresh in memory, the true enormity of four thousand such deaths came pressing down. At the memorial service, scores of faces had flashed by on the video screen along with the captain's. Some I recognized. Most I did not. All these lost lives became familiar, and heavy. It hurt. And that was necessary.

# 12

# It Just Might Work

I DON'T feel comfortable putting him in the VR under the circumstances," Samantha, our newest research psychologist, announced at our weekly meeting.

Three deep breaths, I told myself, practicing a technique we had been teaching our patients. It had been a tense few months. Since Jim's departure, we had been under pressure to get the virtual reality projects running or else lose our funding. After a long delay, we had finally gotten the administrative aspects in order. We had hired therapists, gotten institutional review board approval, done training in virtual reality therapy. Everything was in place, except for the thing we thought would be easy. Patients weren't coming in. Although the media loved the idea of using computer simulations to treat PTSD, those that actually suffered from the disorder found VR therapy less appealing. In the prolonged exposure arm of the study, we had not managed to get a single individual to show up to treatment.

"He wants to do it," I told the research group, trying to convince myself as much as them. "And we already know VR-assisted exposure therapy is a useful treatment modality. You proved that with Virtual Vietnam," I indicated to our collaborators from Virtually Better.

"Yes, but there are a lot of bright lights on us now. Do you think it's wise to have our first treatment subject be someone who came out of the hospital so recently? Think about how it is going to look if something goes wrong," responded Ken Grapp, the head of Virtually Better.

"Half the patients I meet every day are suicidal or just out of the hospital," I said. This high rate of severity was by virtue of my running the emergency team and is not typical of patients with PTSD. My experience with those in crisis, however, told me that this individual could be safely managed as an outpatient. "How about I treat him myself? That way we aren't pressuring Samantha into doing therapy she isn't comfortable with, and if something goes wrong, well, he is already seeing the emergency psychiatrist. We are supposed to be the center of the universe as far as PTSD treatment goes. If we turn him down, who else is going to help him?"

"Well, you're the primary investigator," said Walter, the research assistant who had done the initial assessment on the patient. "I guess you get to decide."

I thought about this for a moment. It was an odd situation. I had not written anything but the smallest sections of the original proposal, but by virtue of my various inherited titles, I was now the head of the project.

"I need to talk to the patient," I said. "Let's see what he wants out of this."

A few hours later I was on the phone with Corporal Philip Spinoza.

"I didn't like being asked all those questions," he said, in reference to the initial exam that had been conducted to see whether he was eligible for the virtual reality treatment.

"It is a very long interview," I sympathized, "but it lets us know the symptoms you are having, and what sort of treatments might best match your needs."

He grunted a rough confirmation of understanding. "So you think this virtual reality stuff is the best match for me?"

"I'm not sure. Judging by the reports I read about you, it seems like an appropriate treatment, but I want to get to know you better first. You ever heard the one that goes, 'How many psychiatrists does it take to change a lightbulb?'"

"Nope. How many?" he said without a hint of humor.

"One, but the lightbulb has to want to change."

"Is there a point to that joke?"

"Well, I'm trying to figure out what you want to change."

"How about all those rules?"

I thought about this for a moment. I had meant for him to identify the symptoms he sought to target, but could we negotiate the way we would do the therapy? Research protocols generally require the patient and therapist to do things in very rigid ways. In this case, a patient entering virtual reality treatments was supposed to agree to come in for appointments twice a week for five to seven weeks, to not engage in other therapy during that period, and to avoid alcohol or tranquilizers.

"Some of those rules are there for us, and some of them are for you," I said. "I won't negotiate on the ones that are there to protect you. That means you can't drink alcohol or use benzodiazepines if you are in the virtual reality treatments. They could prevent the treatment from working. Also, you have to agree to regular assessments."

"More questions?"

"Yes, it's hard to get around that," I said. "I am confident that with or without virtual reality, we can find a form of treatment to help you. What I am not confident of is that whatever we do first is going to be the perfect match. There is always guesswork involved, and the only way for me to know that I am not making you worse is to keep assessing your symptoms. Most important, you have to be able to tell me if you are getting suicidal again, because if you end up dead, that is the one thing I can't go back and fix."

"I can do that. I promised my doctor when I left the hospital that I would let her know if things were getting worse again."

"And have they been?"

"No, but they ain't much better either. These pills haven't done squat."

I looked over his medical record. He had been taking an antidepressant for the last eight weeks. Normally, we would hope to see a response by now, but sometimes it takes longer.

"Have you had any side effects?"

"Nothing at all. It's like I'm taking water."

"Well, medication is one of the things I'm willing to be flexible about," I said. "The reason we have the rules about not changing meds or doing other therapies is that we are trying to figure out what the virtual reality treatment actually does, and it's hard to see that if we keep changing other treatments."

"I haven't really been going to my therapy appointments anyway. I've got work to do, and I don't want to be seen as a slacker."

"I can be flexible on the appointment times too," I said. "The reason for that rule is that we were trying to standardize the treatment so that we can pass it on to other therapists in cookbook form. Since that rule was for us, I'll bend on it."

He was quiet for a moment. Only the sound of deep breathing came through over the line.

"You are on a profile, aren't you?"

"Yeah, what of it?" Spinoza said a little defensively.

A *medical profile* is a category into which the military puts Service Members who are not healthy enough to do their regular jobs but not so sick that they might not recover and get back to work. This is an Army term. The Navy and Marine Corps call it *limited duty*, but it is essentially the same. Conditions such as a broken arm or a bad case of pneumonia are causes for such a designation and so is post traumatic stress disorder. The difference between the situations is that with a broken arm, everyone can clearly see why you aren't carrying your full weight right now. With PTSD, sometimes you have to defend yourself from the accusation that you are avoiding work.

"I'm not accusing you of anything," I explained. "I just thought that it might do some good if I contacted your company commander and let him know that if he let you go for treatment more frequently, it could mean that you are back to full duty all the sooner."

You could hear the pain and conflict in the corporal's voice as he responded to this offer. "I don't know," he choked. "I want to go back to my unit. I really do, but I can't do it. I can't be around them right now. I don't see how I'm ever supposed to go back to the range."

"You will," I reassured him. "I don't want to lie to you. This therapy is new. You will be the first individual that I have personally treated with it. If the textbooks are right, it is going to be hard as hell, but the book also says that the harder you push yourself, the better your chance of success. There are no guarantees, but if you want to go back to being an artilleryman, I'll work with you as hard as I can to get you there."

"I ain't trying to do nothing less."

We talked for another hour on the phone. Spinoza told me about what had happened to him in Iraq and how he had changed since he got back. Not every Service Member who has PTSD is motivated to return to his or her unit, but Spinoza definitely was, and I took that as a good sign. We looked at the things he was doing in his life that were already helping him and the stuff he knew wasn't so healthy. He agreed to a plan to try to accentuate the positive. In the meantime, we would meet and talk.

The next day we met in my office. He was shorter in real life than he had sounded on the phone but no less a Soldier. I started off by explaining how we would approach treatment and the reasons I would be pushing him to face his difficult experiences. The therapy would proceed at his pace, and he could say stop at any point. In general, however, I was going to be encouraging him to face things that were distressing. To facilitate monitoring as we went along, we would use a scale called Subjective Units of Distress, or SUDs. This put a percentage rating on how uncomfortable he was at any given moment. Zero meant that he was in no distress at all, and one hundred indicated that right now was the worst moment of his life. In each session, we would aim to make things a little uncomfortable, say, a SUDs of about fifty to seventy. Then we would keep working on that same issue until we found that it was easier, that his SUDs rating dropped. Sometimes the SUDs might decrease at the end of a story. Other times, we might have to work on it over and over again.

I asked him to repeat the same story he had told me over the phone, about what happened to him in Iraq, but to also imagine himself there and to tell the story as if he were narrating a movie he was watching right now. He hesitated briefly, but like a good Soldier, he launched in as instructed. It was obviously rough for him.

"OK. On that zero to a hundred SUDs scale, how are you doing?"

"About a sixty."

"So, it is more difficult this time than the first?" I asked.

"Yeah." I could tell he was doubtful about how treatment had started off.

"That's OK," I explained. "You are actually doing really well. It is not uncommon that in telling a traumatic story it gets harder before it gets easier. Remember, if it is too much, we can stop, but I really would like you to go through it again if you can."

He did, and this time he reported that it was a little better, not a lot, but a little.

"This isn't fun, Doc."

"I know, and I realize the tremendous effort it takes on your part to face these things. Also the trust that you are placing in me that this is actually going to help. I really appreciate your effort."

He took a deep breath and went at it again. About an hour and a half later, we stopped.

"Pretty messed up story, huh, Doc?"

"It is. War is messed up. I didn't think you had PTSD from an event that wasn't horrific. We will deal with it."

We chewed the fat a while longer, just talking now. It was time to cool down, to talk not about his experience in Iraq but his experience here.

"And how are you doing now?"

"SUDs are all washed out," he smiled. It was the first time I had seen him do that.

"It's good to laugh if you can," I said. "I'm a big believer in bad joke therapy."

"Stick with that lightbulb one then. It's a stinker."

It was my turn to crack a smile. I had some serious issues to address, though.

"Any thought about hurting yourself?"

"None. And no thoughts toward hurting anyone else, either." He anticipated my next question. "I know I'm not going back to that dark place again, and if I do, I'll call."

"Good. Now we do have homework to assign. We only have so much time together, so you need to continue the work between sessions."

"OK, what do I have to do?"

I handed him a cassette tape. "I want you to listen to yourself," I said. "This does two things. First, it lets you keep working on that habituation thing we talked about. Second, it lets you put a more objective spin on things. You seem pretty hard on yourself. I want you to think about how this story sounds, objectively, if you really think that you have anything to feel guilty about, or if anyone in your position wouldn't have done the same thing."

He seemed uncomfortable with the idea, not quite ready to forgive himself for what had happened. But he took the tape.

"There's more?" He asked with the expression of a high school student being told to write term papers over his spring break.

"I know this is a pain, but we only have a few hours together a week. If you really want to accomplish something, it is important to be spending most of your waking hours working toward that goal. This is no exception. The second area I want you to keep working on is to challenge yourself toward getting back to the range."

He shook his head vigorously. "I told you, I ain't ready for that, Doc."

"I know," I said, spreading my hands in what I hoped was a calming gesture. "I'm not asking you to do it right away. It is just so you know where you are headed. What I want to do before you leave today is identify three areas of your life where you have been avoiding things, things that you have to face up to in order to get back into your regular life: going to restaurants, talking to your buddies again, being around loud noises. Each is a step that gets you closer to the artillery range. Even for these smaller tasks, you don't have to face them all at once. I want you to outline steps that would build up to it. For example, you don't have to go into the restaurant the first time. You can just stand outside. The one thing I don't want you to do, though, is back out once you have started facing an uncomfortable experience. Pick something you can tolerate, and then work your way up to it."

"So standing outside a restaurant is all I have to do?"

"To start," I said. "Keep pushing yourself. In particular, I want you to keep pushing yourself back into talking to people. I think I'm a pretty good doctor, but if you can talk to the people who were there with you, or those who know and love you, I think they will be better than I, or any other professional therapist."

Spinoza wrote down a list of tasks to accomplish and specific dates to set a time line. I was impressed with his willingness to move forward, even though this all sounded crazy to him.

The next week he came in with a neatly printed log of his accomplishments for the week.

"There is spaghetti sauce on the last page," he noted, without a visible display of humor on his face.

"You made it inside the restaurant?" I nodded, impressed.

"It wasn't what I call a fun meal, but yeah, I did it."

"Good. Excellent. And how distressing was it?"

"About a fifty," he said, using the numeric shorthand we had developed through the first session.

"OK, that is the range of stress we want you to be tolerating. We will talk about more homework at the end today, but for now I want to introduce you to the virtual world."

He grew visibly tense. In later patients this would become something that was quite familiar. Often the most distressing aspect of virtual reality is the idea of going into it. At that point, I was tense myself. Up until now, the therapy was the same as we would have used in traditional prolonged exposure. We were both about to venture into the unknown.

"SUDs now?" I asked.

"Let's just say it's high. Give me the goggles before I change my mind."

Spinoza was now in the same chair in which I had sat when Dr. Spira had put me into Virtual Iraq. I hooked him up to wires and connectors and then cranked up the computers. He wore a set of virtual reality goggles that adjusted the view as his head and body moved in space. Headphones piped in the sounds of the car and desert. His chair was sitting on what we called a "vibration platform," which was really a giant subwoofer pumping out the low-rumbling feel of a Humvee. To his left was a smell machine, capable of producing the odor of diesel fuel, or of gunpowder or blood, as the situation merited. We didn't use the smells yet, and unlike my first experience in the machine, we kept the scenario peaceful. There would be no ambush today and hopefully no computer glitches.

Spinoza steered through the desert simulation using a game controller similar to what you would find on a PlayStation or an Xbox. On my desk were two other computer screens, one of which showed what he saw through the goggles. The scene shifted as he turned his head to the left or right. The second screen was the control interface. On this monitor were a collection of menus, allowing me to pick everything from the time of day, to the weather, to the level of violence going on in the background or near the Humvee.

"How are you doing now?" I asked through the microphone that was plugged into his headphone system.

"NOT TOO BAD!" He yelled back. One of the side effects of the VR sound system is that people often speak as if they were really in a noisy Humvee, forgetting that the world outside is actually an otherwise quiet doctor's office.

"Good. I want you to drive around for a while. Let me know when you get comfortable."

He passed by the same statue and overpass where I had experienced my virtual ambush. No floating figures appeared. The software guys had been doing their work.

"I THINK I'M READY, DOC," he said, in a volume that was nearly deafening. I reminded myself to ask about extra insulation for our room so we would not disturb doctors down the hall.

"Good. I'm going to make things a little more stressful, if that is OK with you."

Spinoza nodded.

"We will start by changing it from day to night, since the experience we will be working on happened at night."

I clicked the menu controller, and the blue skies shifted to a star-filled firmament. Shadows filled the screen.

"IT'S TOO DARK. WE HAD NIGHT VISION," Spinoza protested.

"OK, I think I have an option for that." I pushed another button and a brighter, but green-tinted hue took over the monitor. "How are you doing now?"

"ABOUT A FIFTY."

"Good. Let's stay with that until you start to feel more relaxed here too; then we will add a few more elements."

Not too much later Spinoza again nodded his readiness to advance in the scenario.

"OK, this time I am going to add a sound that is specific to the story you told me yesterday. There is going to be the sound of artillery off in the distance, but only off in the distance. Are you ready?"

"SIXTY PERCENT STRESS, BUT READY."

I turned up the external speakers in the room so I would know when the sounds came through and then moved the cursor over the button for the sound of distant gunfire.

There was a low rumbling boom, and Spinoza flinched in his chair—the familiar, exaggerated startle response of a patient with PTSD.

Spinoza settled quickly. "I'M FINE. YOU CAN DO IT AGAIN," he said after a few minutes of intervening silence.

I fired off the simulated artillery again, and once more Spinoza flinched, although not as dramatically as with the first blast. We repeated this same exercise a dozen or more times before our hour ended.

"You did really well," I said as the time came to remove the headsets. "Next session we are going to bring it all together. You are going to tell your story the same way you did the first time, but while driving the Humvee, the way you did today."

Spinoza looked exhausted, but as before, he took the tape of the therapy session and agreed to a series of tasks in which he would challenge himself between sessions.

I was concerned when he canceled our next appointment. I called him at home.

"Are you doing OK?" I asked.

"Not too bad, but I'm busy this week. Maybe we should put things off for a while?"

I was in a dilemma about what to say next. This was a critical juncture. With any anxiety-provoking therapy, there is the possibility of making patients worse before they get better. Spinoza had already had a hard time connecting with a therapist. If I drove him away now, he might never get into the treatment he needed. How could I get him to come back? Avoidance is one of the main symptoms of PTSD, but people have legitimate reasons for missing sessions. Spinoza had also previously demonstrated that other quintessential symptom of PTSD, irritability. I wanted to challenge his resistance to treatment, but I had to do so without driving him farther away.

"Well, do you want to reschedule for a particular time next week?"

"I'll call you," Spinoza said in a flat tone.

"You do realize that if you don't I'm going to keep bugging you, don't you?"

"Hey, Doc, I know it sounds like a blow off, but I really will call. I just have some things I need to work out with my wife first."

"Why don't you bring her in," I offered. I realized I should have asked this sooner. PTSD never exists in a vacuum. It can have tremendously devastating effects on families and marriages. Conversely, having a good family support system, especially one that encourages the PTSD sufferer to stay in treatment, can make the difference between failure and recovery.

"I'll have to ask her about it," Spinoza said, still doubtful.

"How about next Wednesday? I think you told me that was her day off."

"Yeah, I'll ask."

The intervening week was not without anxiety, but on Wednesday at 0900 hours Mr. and Mrs. Spinoza arrived exactly on time. Her name was Maria, and given her angry countenance, I had to remind myself not to associate her with the PTSD patient with the same first name.

"Thank you for coming, Mrs. Spinoza."

"I suppose you are going to give me a bunch of excuses for how Philip has been acting, saying it isn't his fault?"

"Well, if it is OK with both of you, I'd like to get a better picture of what is going on."

"Why should we have someone else there just for us to talk? We never used to need that."

"Perhaps, but you have bigger problems now, and sometimes big problems require you to schedule time to work on them. Having a mediator can help to make sure that things move along and can also give you a stop time so that any one discussion doesn't become overwhelming."

Maria Spinoza continued her scowl, but it was obvious by the way she was looking at her husband, that she cared about him very much. "I'll do it if he will," she said.

Corporal Spinoza nodded in agreement also.

"Good, now, while I have you here, Mrs. Spinoza, I want to touch on something you said earlier, about excuses and this not being Philip's fault."

"Go on. I knew this was going somewhere."

"Well, it is true that what happened to your husband is not his fault. I am not making excuses, however. Taking care of it is his responsibility."

"What's the difference?"

"Well, if you had the flu, and threw up on the floor, that wouldn't be your fault. You didn't ask to get sick, and it definitely wouldn't help for someone to be mad at you for being sick."

"So you are saying I am wrong for being mad?"

"Not necessarily. If you had thrown up on the living room carpet, that is not your fault. But it also isn't anyone else's. It was your mess, and it is your responsibility to clean it up. People might be justifiably upset if you left it there."

"It might be nice if someone helps out, if I'm sick."

"True, and that is what I would ask that you do for your husband. Help him out. But, for you, Philip, I would ask that you understand that your wife does not owe you this. It is your responsibility to take care of yourself and the problems you cause."

They both tentatively agreed. I explained to Mrs. Spinoza about the symptoms of PTSD and the reasons for the therapy. I asked that she help in making sure that her husband did his homework between sessions and showed up to the next one.

Two days later Corporal Spinoza was back in my office and seated in the VR simulator.

"That was a dirty trick, Doc," Spinoza said, but again he was smiling. "You knew that my wife ain't ever going to let me out of showing up."

"I had my suspicions. Did she get you to do your homework as well?"

"Yeah, we've been doing the whole thing, going to couples counseling, going to restaurants. She even listened to the tape with me one time, and she didn't freak out."

"And you?"

"It was difficult, but I made it through."

"Good. Are you ready to start today?" I asked.

He was nervous, but proceeded. I started up the simulation of the Humvee, and he began driving along the road. This time he narrated from his memory, and I did my best to match the simulation to what he was describing.

"It was dark," he said. "Because of all the dust kicking up, we couldn't see much of anything, even with the night vision. I was driving the second Humvee, and there were three guys with me. Chancy was supposed to be in the turret, but he never could see squat in the dark, so we let Bills take his shift."

I watched Spinoza's breathing start to increase. "You are doing well," I said. "How is your stress level?"

"About a fifty-five," he said, and continued with his story.

The number increased as his narration went on. I kept the additions mild for this session. For now, I let him talk about explosions without adding the simulated versions. There was enough going on in his mind. At times, he even closed his eyes, lost in the memory of his worst day. I had not turned on the smell machine, but Spinoza described the scent of gunpowder and sand as the ambush began.

"I knew something was wrong as we came under the overpass. That car up there was moving too slow. I was going to tell Bills to keep trained on it, but I thought he had it. Bills was always on the ball, except for that day."

"You are doing great, but tell it as if it were going on right now."

The world on the screen shifted up and down as Spinoza nodded understanding. For him, the world would appear stable, matching the image to the movements of his head. He continued on for about ten minutes before we came to the hardest part of the story. Spinoza took a deep breath in preparation.

"I'm not sure if I heard the shot that hit us. There was so much fire going on, but then all of a sudden the windshield burst. Then there was this fine, pink mist everywhere. I couldn't tell if it was blood at first, because, since I was wearing the night goggles, I could only see the color in my peripheral vision. Then it started spraying out of Chancy in bursts. I turned to my right and a chunk of his neck was missing. An RPG had hit us dead on. The fin had sliced right through Chancy, and the grenade lodged in the back seat. It hadn't exploded."

"I know this is really hard to tell, but you have done very well." I tried to reassure him. "How are you doing now?

"About a ninety-five," he said, a quaver in his voice. I backed down on the sound effects and just listened to his voice as he continued. "I hit the gas as hard as I could, trying to get out of there, though we were carrying the ordinance. Chancy wasn't dead yet, and blood was everywhere. It made the steering wheel slippery. In the meantime, Bills must have spotted the shooter on the overpass because he opened up with the fifty cal. Parts of the roadwork started falling down, and I think I saw a body, though it was hard to tell. We definitely hit something in the road as we passed under, and I was sure the damn RPG was going to go off."

Spinoza finished telling the story, winding down with his escape, his efforts to remove the body of his dead friend from the vehicle all the while wondering if he shouldn't abandon him because of the un-exploded rocket that still lodged in the damaged vehicle. It seemed like he wasn't quite sure where the story would end. The whole day was relevant. How could he leave any of it behind? Then, abruptly, he cut into his own story.

"I guess that's it," he said. "I'm done."

I clicked off the video simulation, and let him remove the headset. He looked shaken.

"How was it?" I asked.

"Not fun, but not as bad as I expected. The video and sound did make it more real. It reminded me of things I had forgotten, but maybe I needed to remember."

"The idea that therapy should reveal the unconscious goes all the way back to Freud," I said. "I'm not sure what he would think of your experiences in the VR, but I was very impressed with how you handled them."

"I guess I'm supposed to do it again now?"

"Yes, I know it's hard, but that is how it works."

He repeated the story more that day, and more in our next several sessions together. Each time we focused on the most difficult sections for him, going over them until they lost their power. Also, we made the VR a little tougher. I never got the smell machine working properly, but, at the right times, I tried to open the vials that smelled like gunpowder smoke. The platform shook with the explosions, and each time, he flinched less. Then, in the fifth session, he surprised me.

"I think I'm ready to go back to my unit, Doc," he said. "I think I'm over it."

Again I was on the horns of a dilemma. This was, after all, what we were aiming for. I very much wanted him to be better. It was good for him, and looked good for my research. One of the first things they teach you, both as a psychiatrist and as a scientist, is to be wary of accepting an idea too quickly, especially if you know that your own biases are going to make you want to accept it. It would be easy to declare victory and go home, but it crossed my mind that this might all be a more byzantine form of avoidance. Since he now knew that his wife was going to make him keep coming as long as he had PTSD, wouldn't the most effective way to avoid treatment be to claim that he was cured?

"Well, 'over it' can mean different things," I said. "Do you mind if we go through that annoying testing again? I want to make sure that I'm not missing anything."

"No problem, Doc."

I started down the checklist of the seventeen symptoms of PTSD. Sure enough, he reported improvements in all areas. More important, he didn't report unrealistic improvements. Anyone who comes back from war is going to have some bad feelings associated with the experience. If he was lying about his symptoms improving, he was at least doing an effective job of making it look real.

I also repeated the checklist questions about depression, physical complaints, and general anxiety. Once again, he reported improvements in areas where he had previously shown impairment. The changes were not as dramatic as they had been for his PTSD symptoms. For example, he claimed no improvement at all in the back pain that had been plaguing him but said that he worried about it less now. He appeared to be showing a collection of symptoms that, although not gone altogether, would no longer be considered diagnostic in any category. Simply put, he no longer had PTSD.

Of course, the tests were only as good as the answers he gave, and I was not fully convinced.

"I'm glad you are doing better," I said. "But going back to your unit would be a very big step. Sometimes people have good periods and bad periods. Why don't we see if your improvement holds up if we make things a little more stressful today?"

"Fine by me," he said and launched easily into the narrative that had previously caused him so much trepidation.

I didn't hold back in the VR. As he talked about explosions, I simulated explosions. As he talked about blood, I brought in the sounds of screaming and pain. He kept talking. He was quite calm, not without emotion, but what you might expect from someone telling a horrific tale that was also true. It was painful but not debilitating.

When we finished that day, I was impressed.

"That was incredible," I said. "What do you think allowed you to make this sudden turn around?"

He shrugged. "Different things. I don't want to knock what you did for me here, Doc, but a lot of it was that I finally decided to stand up. Also, I started talking to my wife, and she helped out."

"That makes sense to me," I said. There is research in psychology that suggests that it is as much the decision to come to treatment as the therapy itself that results in improvement. Later work would convince me that, at least in chronic PTSD, the form of therapy really does matter, but for this first case, the recovery seemed too miraculous to be attributed to a few sessions in a simulation.

"So, do I get to go back?" he asked.

I was still cautious. "Not yet," I said. "This is just one session. Let's see if your improvements hold up. I want you to come back next week, and we will run you through the simulation again, and I'm going to throw the kitchen sink at you. If you do OK in the VR, I'll send you back to my research assistant for another full assessment. We can go from there."

In the intervening week, I boned up on all the ways stress could be introduced into this particular simulation. There was an ambush, a sandstorm, many events that had nothing to do with his individual trauma, but which, if he were eventually returned to his unit, or God forbid, Iraq, he might have to face without cracking. None of this changed the outcome. He admitted that Virtual Iraq was still not a walk in the park, but he responded appropriately to all the situations. He performed as a Soldier should perform.

The final assessment showed a few ongoing problems, some of which had not appeared when I had gone through the checklist of questions with him.

"Can I ask what has you depressed?" I asked.

"I had more problems with my wife," he said. "It is nothing out of the ordinary. We had these kinds of fights before I went to Iraq. It still gets me down, but I'm not putting a gun in my mouth this time, and I'm ready to go back to my unit."

"OK," I said.

Back he went.

# 13

# The State of the Science

POST traumatic stress disorder has a rule of halves. Only about half of Service Members who develop PTSD after combat will end up in treatment. Half of those who do make it to therapy will receive what the Rand Corporation famously called "minimally adequate treatment." Before virtual reality, the best available therapies generally boasted about a 50 percent success rate. We had to do better. This is what we set out to accomplish with virtual reality treatment.

The bar seemed set pretty low, but it was a notoriously difficult task to achieve. Although the numbers might seem bleak, to many people, 50 percent was an overestimation of the success rate. The success rate for "best practice treatments" was taken from statistics on civilians. Many treatments, including some medications the US Food and Drug Administration approved, had failed to work when tested on Veterans. In the years of the Iraq and Afghanistan wars, the US government poured more than three hundred million dollars into developing new treatments for combat-related PTSD. As of this writing, not a single one of them was shown to be better for combat Veterans than what was already available. Coming up with effective treatments and testing them in combat Vets had both proved to be daunting tasks.

I had the opportunity to work directly with a few patients using virtual reality, but I did not treat most participants in the program. We had a group of excellent research psychologists who worked with patients and the machines: William Deal, Karen Pearlman, Carol Russ, and Dennis Wood. My predecessor, Jim Spira, and my interim replacement while I was in Iraq, Scott Johnston, also used the VR to treat PTSD. It was their work, both the therapists' and the patients', that really made the difference. As supervisor, however, I was blessed with the opportunity to meet these fine Service Members. I'd introduce myself and learn something about their lives.

"Hi, I'm Dr. McLay. I'm the primary investigator on the virtual reality projects. I like to check in with people as they go into the VR treatment and when they leave, so that I can see what is, and is not, working. So, tell me how you are doing?"

We had all types: men, women, nineteen-year-olds who had spent their first year of adulthood under fire, and seasoned Veterans called back from the reserves after many years of civilian life. There were one-, two-, and even three-war survivors. Some had been in reasonably peaceful areas but had been unfortunate enough to hit a particularly bad event. Others had spent their entire deployment under direct fire. Many Service Members had visible scars from the war but more common were invisible wounds. This included not only PTSD but also the other signature injury of the Iraq war, traumatic brain injury (TBI). TBI most commonly occurred during an IED blast in which the modern body armor had saved their lives but not always those of their comrades. Most of our patients had suffered in silence for months—if not years—before coming to medical attention, and for many of them, even when they had sought help, it had been to no avail. Medication, therapy, church, drinking away their problems—nothing had worked. What they had in common was that when they arrived, they were not doing well. All of them could identify something that they wanted to change, something that they wanted to fix within themselves.

To be entered in our studies, a Service Member had to have an existing diagnosis of PTSD that had lasted at least three months. He or she also had to be willing to commit to a very difficult course of therapy and to give up certain crutches, such as alcohol or other intoxicating substances while receiving the treatment. If the individual had been a ground combatant, he had to have tried at least one other form of therapy.

Patients were sent to one of our two VR programs. Frontline combat troops were sent to the more aggressive, prolonged exposure approach. Others, what the Marines call POGs (people other than grunts), were assigned to the more gradual approach that involved relaxation training. All who entered therapy had to work hard and accept that facing something they wanted to avoid was actually going to help them. It was not an easy thing to do, and it tended to give us a motivated group.

Typical of these was Petty Officer Kahn. Kahn was a waifishly thin woman in her mid-twenties. She was a medical corpsman, one of the few females in her unit. She had faced isolation and fear for her own life, and, with only a few months of medical training, she had dealt with what war could do to the bodies of the living and the dead. She did her job while she was deployed, but when she came back, she found the memories were too much for her. She drank, got in trouble, and finally came to medical attention because the officer who gave her the last reprimand realized that this was not the same young woman he had sent to war. He told her to get help, and she listened.

When I first met her, she was fidgeting in her chair and would not make eye contact. "What do you want to get out of this treatment?" I asked.

"I want my life back. I want to be able to do my job. I want to be the person this war took away from me. I'm scared of everything now, and I'm sick of it."

She was assigned to work with Dr. Wood, our most experienced therapist and a retired Navy captain. We had a huge problem with patients not showing up to therapy after their initial interview. As scared as Khan appeared, I was worried that she might disappear. Dr. Wood had a good habit of always meeting with patients as early as possible to keep them engaged. In this case, it certainly worked.

Ten weeks later, I was pleased to find that she had made it all the way to the end of treatment. I was thrilled to see what had changed. All of the symptoms of PTSD had improved, and she also reported that her mood and anxiety were much better than they had once been.

"I'm not saying everything is back to the way it was," she explained. "I still think about the awful stuff I saw. I can't imagine I'll ever think of burning meat in the same way. But I do have my life back. I kept my promise not to drink, which was hard at first, but now seems to be something I can do for the rest of my life. Also, I have one big bit of news."

"Yes?"

"I'm going back to Iraq in a few months. I'd never thought I'd be able to do that."

"And how do you feel about it?"

"I'm not sure. I'm scared, but not in the way I was scared of everything before. I'm proud that I'm able to do it, even though Dr. Wood explained to me that I'll have a higher chance of coming back with PTSD again than someone who never had it."

"No one knows exactly what the risks are in these cases," I said. "We really weren't able to fix people in previous wars."

"But I do think I am fixed, or better anyway. I broke my ankle as a kid, and I know that means it is more vulnerable to breaking again. It's the same—ankle or PTSD. I'm not going to give up running, and I'm not going to give up being a corpsman."

Kahn was among a minority of patients that actually returned to combat. Other issues often meant that the Service Members were leaving the military anyway.

Corporal Yin was a tall, solidly built man, barely old enough to shave, but with a cragged and scarred face that made him look much older. He had undergone a significant head injury when he was blown up by an improvised explosive device. He was being medically retired from the military because of the TBI, and he was often slow to answer questions.

"What do you want to be different?" I asked.

"My sleep," he answered in typical, taciturn style.

"What about your sleep? That you can't get to sleep, or that you have nightmares, or that you don't seem rested when you do sleep?"

"Yeah, that."

Yin worked with Dr. Perlman twice a week for six weeks. Dr. Perlman had had one of the best success records of any of our therapists but hesitated to take on many of the more difficult cases. I had to push her to accept Yin because she had been convinced that his head trauma was too severe for him to benefit from the treatment.

"You might be right," I said. "I'm sure this is going to be more difficult, but he wants to try it, and he doesn't have a lot of other options. Meds didn't work for him, and he isn't exactly the sort who is going to bare his soul in traditional talk therapy."

Dr. Perlman eventually acquiesced. A few weeks later she was beaming at the lab meeting.

"You are going to have to see Yin," she said. "Working with him has been hard because it takes longer in session, but he is a totally different person."

When it came time for the assessment after treatment I noticed something unusual from the scores. His PTSD, mood, and reaction time had all improved.

"So how is your sleep?" I asked, remembering his earlier complaint and wondering whether sleep held the key to other improvements.

"It's much better. I haven't had a nightmare in weeks. Sometimes I still have problems getting to sleep, but once I do, I'm out like a light."

"And you use much longer sentences," I pointed out.

"Yeah, my wife said that too. She asked if you could put that part back the way it was." He laughed.

There has been considerable speculation about the ways traumatic brain injury and PTSD are tied together. It is always foolish to put forth an opinion before all the data are in, but my own contact with these patients had convinced me that these conditions are inexorably linked. We consistently found that, in patients with mild brain injuries, treating PTSD also improved symptoms more traditionally associated with a blow to the head. Memory, concentration, even dizziness or vertigo often improved as PTSD started to resolve. Perhaps it was because of better sleep, but we were always glad to see the improvement.

Traumatic brain injury was not the only issue that clouded the picture with PTSD. Life is messy, and as motivated as our patients were, other issues came up.

"I know I'm better now, but life is still hard," said Lance Corporal Beratelli when I talked to him after he finished treatment. "My girlfriend isn't coming back, and my pay is docked for the trouble I got into before treatment."

"Do you need additional help?" I asked.

"I know I need more help, but not from the virtual reality, and not for the PTSD. I can face what I need to face. I've dealt with what happened in Afghanistan. Now I need to start putting my life back together. It's still a long road back."

We got the lance corporal into financial and relationship counseling as he left our program, but like he said, it was still a long road back.

It wasn't always just the negatives that complicated issues. As strange as it might sound, sometimes there could be too much support.

"I'm not sure what would happen if I got better," Staff Sergeant Walker told me in an interview after he had gone through a round of treatment. "They are putting me out because of the leg injury anyway. The leg is bad enough that I can't do my job as a Marine, but I don't think they are going to give me a very high disability rating for it. The PTSD gets me more disability pay, but now that I've had this treatment, I'm sure they are going to want to reevaluate. The better you make me, the more money I lose."

There has been discussion in the mental health community about compensating people for having PTSD. On the one hand, it is a combat injury, so it would be grossly unfair not to provide financial remuneration just because the wound is to the mind rather than to an arm or a leg. On the other hand, many people question if unscrupulous individuals manufacture their symptoms to gain disability payments. Even worse, the payments might interfere with recovery in those with genuine PTSD because the compensation weakens an individual's motivation to get better.

Staff Sergeant Walker was among the patients who did not recover. Although this was a disappointment, he got us thinking about how we could use the virtual environment, not only as a way of treating PTSD but also for evaluating the validity of symptoms. No one hates the fact that symptoms can be malingered more than the people who truly suffer from PTSD. Even if it is one in a hundred who do such things, it forces the entire patient population into an additional battle. They had to fight the stigma of the disease, and now they also had to face the suspicions of those who thought they might be faking.

The gold standard for assessing PTSD is still listening to what the patient has to say. There is no scan or lab test that can do better than this. The virtual reality, however, added something that was at least more observable. Instead of relying solely on a story in which an individual says he or she jumps at loud noises, the virtual simulator allowed us to actually see how the patient reacted to various situations. Also, we could monitor a patient's heart rate, breathing, body temperature, even the extent of his sweaty palms as he goes through a simulated combat environment. Our project was not about supporting or refuting a person's claim of PTSD, but it gave us some objective observations.

In chapter 12, I mentioned how seeing my first patient, Lance Corporal Spinoza, perform well in the virtual world gave me confidence in returning him to his unit. This was doubly true when it wasn't a patient with whom I had been working directly.

The Navy had come out with an instruction that any individual taking a psychiatric medication needed a written waiver to carry a weapon or to go on deployment. The problem was that the medication had often been started by an entirely different physician, who might now be out of the Navy. The psychiatrist was left to make a recommendation about a patient he or she really didn't know. Most patients we saw were highly motivated to return to their units. But were they ready? Was I, as a psychiatrist, willing to risk my reputation, and, more important, the lives of Service Members with whom the patient would be serving based on such scanty information?

I began running the patients I saw for medical waiver recommendations through a series of computerized tests to assess their reaction time and ability to discriminate among objects. This was to make sure that the medication hadn't dulled cognitive abilities. How to assess performance under stress was trickier. In response to this, I decided to see how individuals performed in the virtual world. It wasn't exactly a field trial, but it did give a sense of how they were doing.

"I have a few things I want you to show me you can do, Master Chief," I told a senior enlisted Service Member who was asking to go back to Fallujah for a third deployment. "You did well on the tests of reaction time and memory. Now we are going to run you through a few tasks in the virtual reality simulator. When you put on the goggles, you will find yourself in a city in Iraq during a battle. About two blocks up ahead on your left is an ambulance with an injured Marine being assisted by two corpsmen. I want you to maneuver through the simulation until you get to that point. Survey the situation, and then come back to your starting point to report. I'm going to try to distract you as you go along. Just react appropriately and accomplish your mission."

Chief put on the goggles and entered the virtual world.

"This is more realistic than I expected," he said craning his neck to the right and getting used to the way the simulation worked. "When do I start?"

"Whenever you are ready," I said.

We didn't have a way of tracking the Chief's real footsteps, so he still had to use the joystick to indicate when he wanted to move forward, but the chief rapidly adapted, moving from covered point to covered point as he proceeded up the urban battlefield. I hit a button on my control panel to simulate a distant explosion. He flinched slightly at the sudden sound, but after looking around to realize that nothing was happening in his immediate vicinity, he proceeded forward. Another button push later, and the attack of rocket propelled grenades (RPGs) was blocking his progress. The chief stayed under cover and fired a few rounds down range before an American attack helicopter chased the insurgents from the area. He then made the last dash to the location of the ambulance and injured Service Member.

"OK, the corpsmen at the scene have the situation in hand, Chief." I broadcast through the headset he was wearing. "You just have to get back to your starting point to make a report so they can medevac out the Marine."

The chief nodded and retraced his steps back to the spot where he had appeared when he originally donned the VR headset.

"You did great," I said as he took off the equipment.

"Yeah, but your injured Marine is out of uniform." He smiled.

I shrugged, confused. I replayed the video capture of the simulation. Sure enough, the video avatar of the Service Member was dressed in Army rather than Marine fatigues. He was, as the chief had said, out of proper uniform.

"I think you are good to go, Chief," I said, and signed his waiver to return to deployable status.

The use of the virtual simulator to assess combat readiness was never part of a formal research project, so I can't really assess how well it worked overall. It was simply the best thing I had available at the time. In the case of treating PTSD, we started to get back solid statistics. We reviewed the numbers right before I went to Iraq.

Our first summation showed that of thirty-three patients who went through virtual reality treatments, twenty-seven, or about 82 percent, showed improvement by the time we were done. These numbers did not tell the entire story, however. Even within our own treatment types, we were seeing dramatic differences. In patients who had gone through the "tough" method of treatment, the version in which they had to recount their own trauma out loud while they experienced the VR, 75 percent of patients had improved so much that they could be considered in "remission." That is, they no longer technically qualified as having a diagnosis of PTSD. With the more gradual approach, in which patients were taught to relax and then apply this skill to working in the simulation, the remission rates were lower. However, more often, patients tended to like, and stick with, the gradual approach. With the "tough" method, half of the patients disappeared before ever entering the virtual reality, leaving as soon as we explained what was involved in the treatment.

"So what did you think helped you before?" I would ask when I met a patient starting the program.

First Sergeant Kimble's blank expression was pretty typical of the responses I had grown used to. "I don't know," he said. "Not much."

Eight weeks later, I repeated the same question. The first sergeant's symptoms were now in remission, and his overall demeanor was much brighter. His answer, though well considered, was still equally vague.

"I knew you were going to ask that," he said. "And I've been thinking about it. I know that it was good that I was talking to Dr. Deal. Beyond that I'm not sure."

"Do you think that the virtual reality itself helped you?"

"I can't say if it did," he answered. "I might have done as well without it. It seems strange that a fancy video game would have cured me."

It seemed strange to me also. I didn't have any doubt that, having been successfully treated, these Service Members were ready to face what was ahead. What I doubted was how much the machines had contributed to their improvement.

Sometimes patients seemed to like the therapy even when they didn't strike us as having had much improvement. This was particularly true when looking at the relaxation training.

"Well, I guess nothing helped my PTSD," answered Petty Officer Ubin, a construction battalion worker to whom I asked the same questions that I had put to First Sergeant Kimble. "But I'm thankful for what Dr. Russ taught me because I learned important skills. I know how to relax now and that serves me in every aspect of my life."

Ubin was considered one of our definitive "treatment failures." He maintained a diagnosis of PTSD despite having gone through not only the gradual VR therapy but also other forms of treatment, including months of intensive residential care at a VA program. Was he overvaluing an aspect of treatment that really wasn't helpful, or were we looking for improvements in areas that were more important to us than to the patients? Was the basic human kindness that Dr. Russ had offered worth more than the technology or the changes in individual symptoms? Was the simple fact that he was in treatment and talking to me a sign that something had gone right? What did that mean for people who were scared off by the thought of entering a VR simulator?

Our success percentages were better than average, but it didn't seem to make virtual reality look that much different than all the other choices that were out there. It was hit and miss. The questions that Dr. Spira and I had discussed in starting this project were still unanswered. What were the right symptoms to target? Was it actually virtual reality that helped patients get better, or was it patients' own motivation to overcome their fear? If we had randomly assigned people between the two forms of VR treatment, would the same differences have appeared? Was it all worth it? We had spent three years and millions of dollars to treat a mere handful of patients. Could the same thing have been accomplished more cheaply and efficiently by putting those resources elsewhere? There are other forms of good therapy.

Our study so far had been one in which all the participants were assigned to receive the same treatment. This is a necessary step to develop a therapy and to prove that it is safe. The problem with this kind of work is that no causal effect can be inferred. Some participants always get better because of the placebo effect. Our results certainly looked better than what was expected with a placebo or even what would have been anticipated with many traditional treatments. But the exact nature of the placebo effect is different in every group of individuals. To really know what is going on, you need to randomly assign individuals to two groups to see whether one treatment is better than the other.

I brought these concerns to my collaborators on our weekly conference call.

"We've already proved what we set out to establish with current design," I argued. "We should try to get some randomized data among the two types of therapy and a control group. Ideally, I'd like that control group to be the same sort of treatment, just minus the VR headset."

"So you want to compare traditional exposure therapy plus and minus the virtual reality?" asked Dr. Difede, a colleague from Cornell, and the person who had first tested virtual reality treatments in survivors of the World Trade Center attacks.

"Yes. We say this is VR therapy. I think it is important to test the necessity of the actual virtual part."

"That would be an active control," she argued, explaining to the group that I was proposing to study our current treatments against another effective therapy rather than against a placebo. We had previously discussed that a true placebo group would be unethical here since there were already proven therapies for PTSD. "You are going to need hundreds of people to participate if you actually expect to be able to prove a difference."

"I know we aren't going to get enough to prove the difference, but I'd like to be able to at least have some idea if it is there."

"Fort Lewis will be starting a new study soon," interjected Dr. Rizzo, the originator of the Virtual Iraq protocol. "We only have nine months left on this work. They have a new, four-year funding stream. Why don't we let them do the comparison between the therapy with and without the machine?"

"OK, but they are only going to be doing one form of the treatment. Right now, we are the only place where we could compare different ways of applying the technology. Shouldn't we at least look at that?"

I knew that there would be resistance on this issue. The two companies involved in the sets of software were fierce rivals, and a few of the
people supporting the different forms of treatment didn't even want to
be in the same room with one another. Surprising to me, it was the team
that seemed to be losing the current comparison, the group from Virtual
Reality Medical Center, that agreed to try out a competition. The other
scientists, those from the Virtually Better Corporation, the University of
Southern California, Cornell, and Emory, who had advocated the more
stringent approach, were vehemently against the idea. In the end, it was
a battle I could not win.

The scientists on both teams were fine people, who did great things
to help our Service Members and to move knowledge forward in the
field. They were, in many cases, more experienced than I in performing
such studies. I do not impugn their motives or their wisdom in blocking
a comparative study. They were probably right in that such a proceeding
would have led to an inconclusive result. That we ended here, however,
left me frustrated and wondering what to do next.

The team from Virtual Reality Medical Center went ahead with a
randomized comparison between their form of VR treatment and traditional talk and medication therapy. That study, however, wouldn't be
completed until after I got back from deployment. The chance of a definitive answer to my questions was even farther off. After all this work,
I really wasn't sure whether I could recommend that a military physician
in the field go to the trouble of procuring a VR system.

I am a believer in the scientific method and in scientific testing. Good
science is the only way to answer questions about medical treatments.
It is a painful truth of modern life, however, that there are difficulties in providing such answers. It takes a team approach, which means
consensus. Even when the scientific team can agree on what they are
going to do, their proposed work must be reviewed by ethics and scientific review committees. Mountains of paperwork need to be generated.
Huge amounts of time and energy must be invested. All of these were
rapidly coming into short supply. Sometimes the questions just can't be
answered.

As I packed my bags for Iraq, I was reminded of an old commercial
about a brand of aspirin. In that ad, a serious and somewhat-frustrated

looking man talks about how there is all this clinical research supporting the use of aspirin for headaches. He said he didn't care about that. In the end, he took the pill and found that it worked for his headache. That was the research he believed.

I can't say I agree with the man's reasoning, but his thinking was looking more attractive. I was a physician as well as a scientist. In the latter role, I hoped to someday provide more definitive answers, but as a doctor, I had more leeway to gain personal experience. As long as a treatment already had been shown to be safe and effective, a doctor may use his or her own clinical judgment for how to apply that treatment. I was free to use whatever treatments with my patients that I saw fit.

I called up Mark Wiederhold, the owner of Virtual Reality Medical Center. "Mark," I said. "I want to take a virtual reality system to Iraq. Would VRMC be willing to lend one to the cause?"

# 14

# Therapy in Foxholes

WHEN the patient has a machine gun with him on the couch, it can change the dynamics of therapy. Corporal Dagon clutched his weapon like it was a child, one that someone was trying to take away from him. He was right about this. Captain Southern and I were about to remove custody of his fully automatic baby.

"It is a temporary restriction," I explained. "Just until we can get you off the Ativan."

"But I'm going to look like a freak," the corporal protested. "They don't even let you in the chow hall if you don't have your weapon. I'd be out of uniform without it."

"I'll talk to your command about the possibility of removing the firing pin but letting you keep the weapon," Captain Southern interjected. "That way no one will be able to tell."

"No one except me and the insurgents. What's the point of being in Iraq if I don't have a weapon?"

"I'm sure they will find something useful for you to do." I nodded as the corporal left the room with a still sullen expression on his face.

I had been in Iraq only a couple of days, and Captain Southern, my predecessor at Fallujah Surgical Hospital, was running me through the nuances of practicing psychiatry in a combat zone. Our medical team experienced the same delays, frustrations, and sandstorms as we made our way into the country. This had been going on since the beginning of the war. Iraq, however, was starting to change.

After a long period of steadily escalating violence, the military situation in Iraq was finally improving. Here in Fallujah, the location of some of the bloodiest fighting of the war, life was now relatively peaceful. Our predecessors had gone through their entire six-months' deployment without a single mortar shell hitting the base, with little military trauma, and, best of all, without a single death. Even at that moment, I think we knew that this luck would not hold.

"Complacency is our biggest threat right now," the captain explained. "I've picked up quite a few patients like Corporal Dagon since I've been here. They come to Iraq just stabilized on medication or with medications started by doctors here in Iraq, but everyone forgets we aren't practicing in the States. We have to manage the complications."

In the case of Corporal Dagon, he had been treated for PTSD with Ativan. This is an effective, albeit short-acting, medication for anxiety. Its use in PTSD under any circumstances is controversial, but we were running into even greater problems with this type of treatment in theater. In my one week of transition working with Captain Southern, we had four incidents in which prescribed drugs such as Ativan and Xanax were stolen or abused to get high. One led to a serious overdose. Even in individuals like Corporal Dagon, who were taking them as prescribed, these medications slow reaction times and impair judgment. Captain Southern had taken a strict stand that anyone taking such a potentially intoxicating medication was not to leave the base or carry a weapon.

Not allowing firearms for someone who used intoxicating medications had been the Navy's policy all along, but the Army and Marine Corps were more flexible on the issue. Since we were practicing at a hospital that treated members of all four of the US military services, we had to figure out some of the rules as we went along.

"For surgeons, a gall bladder surgery is pretty much a gall bladder surgery," explained Captain Southern. "But for mental health, there are going to be all kinds of issues that they didn't teach you about in medical school. This is the first war where we have had the opportunity to use psychiatric meds and therapy at the front, and the nature of that war keeps changing every day. You are just going to have to figure out what works."

That sounded a little bit like what I was doing with the virtual reality system to begin with. Even getting it here had required considerable improvisation. The "portable" system from Virtual Reality Medical Center had been packaged inside a rugged fifty-pound box on wheels. Wheels, unfortunately, do not work well on sand. Now, having dragged the entire mess through the desert, I wasn't sure exactly what to do with it.

Captain Southern explained, "We haven't actually seen that much acute PTSD this go-round. What we see most are depression, generalized anxiety, and marital problems."

"You do marital counseling here?" I asked.

"Yes, actually, we do. There is a video conference system over in the chaplain's office. It doesn't always work, so we do more education about marital coping than traditional couple's therapy, but it is important. The Army Soldiers can be away from home for sixteen months at a time. That's hard on a marriage. Most of the suicide attempts are about someone's spouse leaving. The Soldiers and Marines come out prepared to be shot at, but it is the small things that get you down."

I had experienced some of this myself. Having talked to many of my colleagues about the rigors of being in Iraq, I had come prepared to deal with incoming fire, 150-degree temperatures, and even the hurry up and wait of military transport. In the end, what stressed me most was the paperwork changes. I was told I was going to deploy ten times before I actually was sent, on the eleventh set of orders. The final instructions to leave came just sixteen hours before I had to say goodbye to my family and get on a plane. I had missed most of the training that was supposed to go with deployment. With the sudden change of plan, I hadn't done my taxes or secured a civilian job, which I would need if the orders proved correct. I was going to be out of the military within fifteen days of returning home to the States. I suppose I should have been worried about not knowing how to fire the pistol they gave me, but what really got to me was the thought of coming back and not being able to pay my bills.

"Everything that goes wrong in regular life goes wrong in war too," Captain Southern explained. "It's just more complicated here."

As the previous team left to return to the United States, and I started to get to know my patients better, it soon became apparent that it wasn't just the current stress that made matters difficult. The vagaries of Iraqi communications and uncertainties about the future affected us all, but I was able to sit back and think. I was able to get my life in order. For people who had come over with emotional baggage from previous combat tours, it was much harder.

"You're dealing with a lot," I assured Major DeSanto, an Air Force intelligence officer who came in asking for something to help him relax. He said that his job was overwhelming and that it was keeping him up at night. He complained of the fourteen-hour workdays, seven days a week, and mountains of paperwork.

"It is a lot," the Major agreed. "Too much."

"What I don't understand," I said, "is that this is the same job you had before. It's always been stressful, but you said you didn't have problems with sleep until now?"

"Well, it's different now. I've seen things," he said.

"What sort of things?"

"I can't tell you. It's intelligence work."

"You don't have to give specific details. Just tell me in vague terms what happened."

"It's a war. People die. Bad things happen. I see them. A couple of times, I was involved. I see things now, and they bring up bad memories."

"And you have nightmares?"

Captain DeSanto looked uncomfortable with the question, but he answered. "Of course. Who wouldn't have bad dreams?"

"And you can't talk about what happened?"

"No."

"Or think about it?"

"I try not to."

"And you have had anxiety and insomnia, been irritable, and had problems concentrating for about how long?"

"About a year and a half."

"Which roughly corresponds to your second deployment, during which time you were shot at, saw people killed, and had one of your colleagues die?"

"Yes."

"Doesn't that sound at least a little like that PTSD thing we talked about?" I asked.

The major balked. "I'm in the Air Force. I don't claim to be out there in the ditches taking fire with the grunts. My job is stressful, but I can't call it combat stress. It's the fourteen-hour days that have gotten to me."

The major was not alone. I saw plenty of people who had dealt well with problems before Iraq who were mysteriously now not coping. Even for those who did, it was clear that previous experiences in war changed their view of the world.

"I've seen what a bullet can do to a person," Gunnery Sergeant Grant explained while sitting in my office. "So, physical readiness test be damned, I'm not going running anywhere that has even the remotest possibility of being within the range of a sniper."

I was in an odd position seeing the gunny as a patient. He was our main administrative liaison for the Marine side of the camp. I had worked with him as a colleague for my first two weeks in Iraq. He was always calm, and he laughed loudly and often. He also had been through four combat deployments, three of them in Iraq, one that included the Battle of Fallujah in 2004. A lot of people died in that battle.

"I don't want to scare these young Marines by talking about it," he said, "but it does bother me. I appreciate having the chance to come in here and just spout off."

And I was happy to help in this way. Our informal chats turned into hour-long sessions about once a week. I think he got something out of it. I know Gunny taught me about how a person could cope well with combat stress, particularly the importance of humor. Although enjoyable, sessions with colleagues blurred the lines of the doctor-patient relationship. A psychiatrist is supposed to maintain a cool distance from patients, be their therapist not a friend. I already mentioned that two of my previous patients deployed with me to Iraq. It's hard to know how to draw proper boundaries as a therapist when you eat with, shower with, and are sometimes dependent on the people you otherwise call patients. As the deployment continued, I ended up treating several more of my colleagues.

Just as Gunny left my office after relating a story about the effects of a mortar attack, an explosion shook the building. The irony did not escape me, although this explosion was not as fear-inducing as you might think, since we had gotten somewhat used to the bomb squad blowing up various things inside the camp. This explosion had a rather different sound, but no alarms set were going off, so I kept writing.

Then I heard Gunny calling down the hallway. "Everybody get to the center of the building! That was incoming."

It might have flashed across my mind to question whether Gunny had the hypervigilance of PTSD, the tendency to look for danger when none exists. Clearly, the sights and sounds of war were more likely to bring out those symptoms than a backfiring car at home, even in someone who didn't have all the symptoms of PTSD. As the expression goes, however, it's not paranoia if they really are out to get you. A moment after Gunny sounded the alarm, the siren resounded throughout the camp, indicating that all personnel should take cover.

In the grand scheme of war, this was a minor event. The next day we went out to survey the damage. Luck was on our side. The round had hit about fifty yards from the hospital, in an ideal site—a large, metal storage box, the type carried by eighteen-wheeler trucks. It had mostly contained the blast. The box was filled with scrap materials. A few pieces of shrapnel had pierced the sides and escaped the box, flattening a tire on a Humvee, but otherwise, the rocket had only turned rubble into smaller rubble.

We had gotten off easy, but being shot at does tend to focus the mind. The blast had shaken loose painful memories for Service Members who otherwise had been staying away from mental health services. Business started to pick up.

"I can't sleep," was the most common refrain, so common that I started digging into records from back in the States. When Service Members return from deployment, we ask questions about their mental and physical health. Normally, we would only be concerned if someone has many symptoms; a simple complaint like insomnia might go unnoticed. Sure enough, sleeplessness was the most common complaint in the stateside records. The insomnia had often improved when we checked back on the patients three to six months later, but it was concerning to note that those who had complained of even mild insomnia early on were more likely to have other PTSD symptoms afterward.

It was possible that insomnia really was one of the first signs of PTSD to appear, but I suspected the disorder was multifaceted. I wondered if the insomnia might just be one of the few problems about which it was socially acceptable to visit the psychiatrist. "Oh, nothing happened lately, but I've been having a hard time sleeping with all the noise, and I wondered if you could give me something for it."

The thing was, I didn't want to just give them a pill. I certainly had no moral objection to sleep medications, but it struck me that in a war zone, it might be less than wise to have a substance in your system that prevented you from waking up in an emergency. Also, what if the complaints about sleep were really an entrée for talking about other problems?

I flipped through a few of my old textbooks on the psychotherapy treatment of sleep. Given how well sleeping pills worked stateside, using the therapy method was a skill that had gone a bit rusty for me. It was amazing how many things didn't seem possible in a war zone. I went through the step-by-step guides by which one was supposed to guide a patient to restful slumber:

1. Make sure that where you sleep is quiet and dark. (Tell that to the artillery.)
2. Set a consistent schedule. (Again, not so much.)
3. Don't worry in bed. (Good luck with that one.)

The techniques for relaxation proved popular, however. A company called Stress Eraser donated biofeedback machines, and I started handing those out. Our physician assistant set up a yoga class. Yoga seems a heck of a lot less wimpy when it is taught by a former SEAL. However, everything we were doing had to be modified, tweaked, or adapted to the realities and prejudices of war.

At the suggestion of a psychiatrist who had been in Fallujah previously, I set up a smoking cessation group. This was not only another socially acceptable way to meet a psychiatrist but also nicotine patches actually worked the same way regardless of what country you were in. This also allowed me to circulate and ask about other choice substances abused in camp.

"Seriously? People are snorting computer-cleaning canisters?" I asked incredulously when I was talking to one Marine about popular ways people get high in camp.

"Yeah, it's called huffing," the Marine explained, while I handed out smoking cessation literature. "Cuts off oxygen to the brain and that makes you woozy. A staff sergeant died in a port-a-potty snorting the stuff a few months ago and that scared people off for a while. The brass even considered banning computer cleaners, but with the way the sand clogs up electronics here, it's pretty much mission-critical equipment. That makes it the easiest thing to get, and it doesn't show up on drug tests. I still wouldn't say it's common, but people do use it to get high."

"And alcohol?"

"It's banned of course, but people will get it in the mail from home. Also, we were supposed to get one beer on the Fourth of July, but rumor was that the commanding general decided to give out two for the Marine Corps birthday and used up our yearly quota."

"I heard the locals sell alcohol over the wire as well?"

"In Baghdad, maybe," the Marine shrugged. "In Anbar, we don't let them get that close to our lines. Besides, opium is actually more popular than alcohol in Iraq. The Prophet specifically spoke out against alcohol. Drugs that didn't exist in the sixth century are apparently a gray area."

For the most part, the camp was fortunate not to run into too many problems with people abusing substances. We did run into one strange case in which a Marine kept being brought in for "psychosis."

"I tell you he was acting crazier than a snake's armpit last night," the man's commanding officer explained when he brought him into the clinic the next morning. "He was talking to people who weren't there, and fighting us all off."

"And you are sure he wasn't drinking or using something?" I asked. I had spent three hours talking with this Marine, and he appeared calm, cool, and collected. He seemed smart and had a good sense of humor. None of this fit the picture of psychosis that had just been described as occurring the night before.

Some conditions, such as schizophrenia, bipolar disorder, or a stroke, can cause spontaneous changes in behavior that are odd and sometimes dangerous. In rare cases, people with those conditions can spontaneously recover. However, there are residual, telltale signs. The person will seem "off" in certain ways that are relatively easy for a psychiatrist to spot. The man I had just interviewed was tired, and he admitted to having blacked out; otherwise, he was completely lucid. In the States, coming in loopy one day and then being normal the next is usually explained by drugs or alcohol.

"We have been convoying together for three days," the CO said emphatically. "No one had any packages from home, and we didn't let local nationals anywhere near us."

"His drug test is negative." One of our techs poked his head in to fill us in on the lab results. "His electrolytes labs are messed up, though. Want to keep him for observation?"

"He could have been withdrawing from something that isn't showing up in his system anymore," I guessed. "The worst effects of some substances don't show up until well after we are able to detect them."

"Did anyone notice that he smells like he washed in breath mints?" the tech observed. "Could that mean anything?"

I had no idea, but luckily Captain Cogar did.

"Mouthwash," said our head ER physician.

"Mouthwash?" the Marine's CO and I asked simultaneously.

"Sure. We see it occasionally in bad alcoholics," Captain Cogar explained. "Scope is almost nineteen percent alcohol. Listerine is well over fifty proof. Mouthwash also has all kinds of other compounds that do strange things to your brain when you drink it. In dry counties back home, it's the only thing with alcohol in it that is for sale on a Sunday. I guess the same principle could apply out here, except that Sunday is all year long."

The Marine's squad-mates were dispatched to search his pack and sure enough returned with two empty bottles formerly filled with minty freshness. Faced with this evidence, the Marine confessed. He had been so nervous out on patrol that he had taken to imbibing. It started with just a shot, but things had gone further than he intended the other night.

We evacuated him to a rehabilitation facility, and I was left wondering what I was going to be able to do for men who would rather drink phenol than tell me they were stressed.

It didn't bother me so much that I had missed detecting the mouthwash. I had never had a good sense of smell, so it was just lucky that the tech had detected the odor. What troubled me was that I had spent three hours with the Marine, and he hadn't said anything about how hard things had been for him. I was already not sure I knew what to tell Service Members who came in to talk to me. How was I going to help people if they didn't trust me to tell me their problems?

The Navy has tried to confront stigma by embedding psychiatrists and psychologists with specific units. Rather than stay on bases, some mental health providers traveled with Marines, becoming one of them so that the Marines would be more likely to trust the doctors and listen to their advice.

There are several issues with this. First, as any embedded reporter can attest, traveling with Marines and being a Marine are not really the same things. Second, there is only one psychiatrist for every ten thousand Service Members. A military vehicle typically carries two dozen people at most. A psychologist traveling in that vehicle might get to know those people quite well, but where does that leave the rest? If the doctor is on the move, how do you find the doctor when you need her? Third, once they trust you, what do you tell them? As I already mentioned, physicians in combat zones are already way off the map from what is taught in textbooks and medical school. Even if the knowledge is adapted for combat, that knowledge is still about treating people in clinics and hospitals. What does a psychologist who spent eight years at a nice, safe university have to tell a veteran of six combat deployments about managing combat stress?

Nevertheless, there is clearly the need for both providers who are down in the trenches and for those who can function in a traditional role. We have to overcome the stigma so that people feel they can trust us, while still maintaining clinics where we can apply our medical knowledge. In Fallujah, we used the divide-and-conquer strategy for these tasks. Dr. Barnum, the psychologist on our team, and Petty Officer Wahl, her assistant, went out on convoys. They traveled out twice a week in an MRAP armored vehicle that was nicknamed the "Shrink Wrap." Petty Officer Delphin and I stayed in Camp Fallujah and tried to run a regular clinic. Dr. Barnum got to know some of the Marines a lot better than I did. She was the first in our unit to earn the Fleet Marine Force pin, an award for working with, and acquiring knowledge of, the Marines. I saw more patients than she did each day. Which of us was doing more good? I don't know.

The differences in our approaches varied more than whether we went on convoys. Dr. Barnum was a psychologist. She had a doctorate in how to do psychotherapy. I was there as a psychiatrist. I had gone to medical school and then residency, training with both psychotherapy and prescribing medications. I used a lot of technology; she mostly used traditional talk treatments. I had spent most of my life around academics. Dr. Barnum was married to a Marine. I was older. She was younger. I was a man. She was the first woman psychologist to fill the mobile mental health position. Our approaches, our temperaments, the tools we could offer our patients, they varied.

"Which one of you should I see?" said a confused-looking lance corporal who came into the space between our plywood offices.

"I think I'm next up," I said, looking at the roster for the day.

The Marine looked puzzled. "It's not set up a particular way?"

"In some cases," I explained. "But most of the time, we start off and just try to figure out what you need. It may turn out that it is one of us, or both of us, or neither. Maybe you will leave here with us setting you up with the chaplain service or a few lab tests. Everyone needs different things while they are serving at war."

It turned out that the lance corporal had been getting teased in his unit, a lot of salty and sexualized language, not an uncommon occurrence in the military. Most Marines would have considered this a small matter when compared with the stress of enemy gunfire. They even might have said that this fraternal bonding was what let them face the daily rigors of Iraq. But this particular Marine had been sexually abused as a boy. For him, the taunts were not friendly. They were far more distressing than terrorists or the separation from home.

It was less embarrassing for him to talk to a man, so he stuck with me for therapy. This may have been important. It was very possible, however, that he could have benefited as much or more from working with Dr. Barnum. Similarity is not everything in treatment. During the course of our meetings, he asked if I had ever been through anything like what he had.

"No," I said. "I have lived a very blessed life, and my childhood has nothing to compare to what you went through. Even if I had, I am never going to be able to see what you see behind your eyes. Although we are different, I still think I can help you get through this."

As I gave that speech, I realized that I was also reflecting on the differences between being seen by a therapist like Dr. Barnum, who was out on the convoys, and by a provider like me, who stayed on the forward operating base It was also the difference between a psychologist who went on convoys and another Marine who participated in the firefight. Each was one step removed from the experience of the patient who needed help. Sometimes people needed to talk to a person who had similar experiences. Sometimes they don't.

It was about a month into our deployment before we started seeing people whose issues actually had to do with combat. Perhaps it had taken those convoys and that trust to start to bring them in.

"So are you going to start using your virtual reality?" Dr. Barnum asked one day after returning from a trip to Ramadi. She had seen me drag the contraption across the sand and had been at a talk I had given about our success with the treatment stateside. It was almost three years since we had put the first patient through the treatment, and things were still going well, both for him and for the treatment. Most people who had gone through our VR programs in the United States had ended up getting better. Like everything we were doing in combat zones, however, it was still unclear if treatments that worked in the controlled world of a San Diego hospital would succeed in the heat and chaos of Iraq.

"I want to make sure that we are matching the right people with the right form of treatment," I said. "I don't want to desensitize Marines for whom it is still healthy to be jumpy at the sound of gunfire."

"I've been doing traditional exposure therapy with a few patients, and so far that hasn't been a problem," Dr. Barnum said. "Get their reactions back to normal; they will still be plenty jumpy."

I nodded. "That's true. Both of us certainly jumped the first time those rockets went off next to the barracks." Dr. Barnum and I had both rushed into the hallway from our rooms when outgoing fire woke us to the reality that we were in a combat zone.

"How much do you think the virtual reality is going to add, considering how much real reality we have going on all around us?"

"That's the part I don't know. Now that you mention it, I do have an Air Force officer who is in an admin position. He's been reluctant to accept that his symptoms might be PTSD, but he might benefit from some computer-simulated prompting to make him realize why he can't sleep."

"I guess you can see what works for him."

"That's what we're always doing out here, isn't it?"

# 15

# The War at Home

$S$USAN Papadopoulos does not have PTSD, nor do her children, but they are all suffering from it. When Susan's husband came back from Iraq in 2004, he was a changed man. Now he had left to go to war again.

"It seemed like a good idea at the time," Susan explained about her husband's departure. "We had gotten to the point where we were afraid to have him at home. He was screaming all the time, and drinking. He had all these rules. The doors and windows had to be locked and checked. Even the mailman wasn't allowed near the house. Bill bought an extra mailbox to put at the edge of the yard, and then when the mail did come, we had to wait an hour before we could check it. We thought that if he could just go back to Iraq, he might figure all this out."

"Was it better when he left?" I asked. Susan had come in for an appointment, she told me, to figure out if she suffered from the adult form of attention deficit disorder. So far, I had determined that she was distracted, but it did not seem as though she was the one with a classic diagnosis.

"For him, I don't know. It might have been better," she said. "From his first few e-mails, I thought he was doing well in Iraq. At least deployment makes him stop drinking. But then he stopped calling. We don't

know if he can't call or doesn't want to. We all miss him so much. The
kids are scared, and I'm worried. What if he comes back worse? What
if he doesn't come back at all? We've been through deployments before,
but now it's like it is one time too many."

Susan was in her late thirties but looked older right now, and tired.
She still had the proud bearing of a woman who had long held the difficult job of military spouse.

Even when a Service Member doesn't have PTSD symptoms, military
life is hard on families. According to a 1992 study, before we were at
war, 90 percent of Army personnel were separated from their families for
at least one night every six months. More than 30 percent of personnel
were away from home for at least a month. For members of the Navy and
Marine Corps, six- to nine-month "floats" to maintain maritime readiness have always been commonplace, but assignments had now shifted
from seaborne missions to ground deployments in combat zones. For a
time, the Army was doing eighteen-month combat deployments to Iraq
and Afghanistan. They returned to twelve months partly because of the
problems families experienced when soldiers were gone for this long.
Servicemen and servicewomen tend to marry younger than their civilian counterparts, and many marriages are built on a cycle of leaving and
returning home. Some families adapt well to it. Others do not.

"You said you've been through some of this before?" I reflected. Susan
had told me that this was Bill's second trip to Iraq, but that she and her
three children had packed his bags for deployment at least six other times
during his military career.

"Every time away has been hard," she said. "It affected the kids differently at different ages. When they were babies, they would get fussier
after Bill left. Angela, my youngest, even stopped eating for a while. It
might have been because the routine was changed. Who knows? She
started eating again, and the pediatrician said not to worry about it, that
kids of all ages have more physical complaints when a parent is gone.
When the kids were a little older, toddlers, I noticed that they took their
cues from me. If I was stressed, they were stressed too, but if I could put
on a strong face, it seemed normal to them. Now that they are in school,
they make up their own minds. Bill used to be good about talking to the
kids before he deployed. The last time he went on a ship's tour, Brian,

our middle one, who was seven at the time, asked if Daddy was leaving because he was mad. Bill said no, and sat him down with a map showing where he was going, and talked about what was special about each place, and what Brian might want him to bring back from there. That really helped. The boys miss their father more, I think. They seem to get more depressed about it. Angela worries."

"You've talked a lot about the kids, but what about you? How did his deployments affect you?"

"What affects the kids is usually what affects me. Even this deployment is that way. Brian's teacher said he might have ADHD, so I thought I might have it too. His psychiatrist wouldn't give him any pills either."

"Reasonable, but you are ducking the question. How did you feel during your husband's earlier deployments?"

"It went in phases, I suppose. When we knew it was coming, there was this anticipation. How was it going to go this time? What did we need to get done? Bill would have extra training before deployment, which meant less time for me, just when I really wanted more of his attention. We would fight, and make up, and fight again. Getting ready to go was always the biggest emotional roller coaster. Then, Bill would leave, and I would be sad and cry, feel guilty for all the fights we had, and then be angry at him for leaving me to begin with. Then I'd feel guilty all over again for being mad. A few weeks or months into it, I'd usually settle down."

"What do you mean by settle down?"

"The kids and I would get into a routine. In the old days, we would wait for a letter or phone call when Bill was in port. Sometimes I'd worry about the port calls. You hear things about the Philippines or Thailand. I trust him though."

The possibility of infidelity is often a concern for both Service Members and their spouses during deployment. There are no official statistics, and certainly it does happen, but military spouses are protected in ways that their civilian counterparts are not. Adultery is a prosecutable offense under the Uniform Code of Military Justice.

"Trust is important to maintain in a relationship, especially during a deployment," I agreed.

"That's just it. Bill doesn't seem to trust anyone anymore, even me."

"We'll get into that," I said. "But first, I'd like to hear a bit more about how you dealt with deployments before your husband went to Iraq."

Susan nodded. "In the old days, we would have to wait for letters or calls. The Internet has helped a lot. After we went through it a few times, deployment seemed normal, a regular part of life. It was hard when he was gone during the pregnancy of our oldest, though."

I made a mental note to ask about depressive symptoms later. Rates of postpartum depression are higher when a spouse is deployed during pregnancy. For unknown reasons, this increased risk seems to persist even if the husband is able to return for the birth and stay to help take care of the child. Just having been away increases the risk.

"About a month before it was time for him to come home, I'd start getting excited," Susan continued. "Sometimes I'd be nervous or conflicted because I knew that I'd made changes around the house that he wouldn't like."

"And when he did come home, did you fight?"

"Not at first. We joke that we've had eight honeymoons, our first and then seven times when he's come home from deployment. It really was like another honeymoon. We'd both be eager for sex but then realize that it took a while to get it right."

"That's very normal," I said.

"Well, after a little while the honeymoon was bound to end. Money and the kids, those were what we would usually fight about. Things would change while he was away, and that would be hard for him."

"I'm sure it was hard for you too."

Susan sighed. "It was. I understood where he was coming from. Bill had been putting his life on the line, and visiting third-world countries. It was hard for him to hear me complain that we couldn't afford rollerblades for the kids. But it was frustrating. Bill expected that since he couldn't spend money or have a lot of fun during the deployment, that now he was entitled to go out and spend and party."

"Did the drinking start with other deployments?"

"Not like it did when he got back from Iraq. Then he was drinking nonstop. When he came back from other places, it was just one or two too many."

"The alcohol would negatively impact the family, though?" I asked. The seeds of alcoholism can start early and be subtle. If alcohol is the way you relax, it can be an easy crutch to lean toward if you get overwhelmed. Family is often one of the best indicators that the crutch has become unhealthy. If a person neglects his wife and children in order to drink, that's a problem.

"Bill would want to go off and party, which would make me feel neglected. We would end up fighting, which he said made him want to get out of the house even more."

"Would this cycle end eventually?" I asked.

"Eventually. It was like when he left. There would be an emotional roller coaster at first, but finally we would settle into a routine. Sometimes his friends would out-and-out tell him that he needed to stop partying and get back to us. It helped if the families of the crew knew each other."

The dynamics of how a unit handles a return home can have a huge impact on families. Units that schedule family-friendly events for homecomings can shift the focus away from unhealthy coping habits, such as drinking, and can build strong, natural support groups. This can be particularly important for individuals such as husbands of female Service Members or families that live off base, where social networks that otherwise bring military spouses together may not be present. Even for the single Service Members, having a unit-wide barbecue or baseball game can help build a larger "military family" that can help when things get hard.

"So deployments were always a cycle of ups and downs for you, but it sounds like that since your husband came back from his first deployment from Iraq, it has been different."

Susan shook her head emphatically. "Much more difficult. Bill is a good husband and father, but one bad day can outweigh a week of good ones. I don't know why he changed. I don't know what to do for him."

Individuals with PTSD can feel like they can never let loved ones know what happened. They think that knowledge is too horrible. It is never easy to hear that someone you love has been traumatized, but often not knowing is even worse. Family members are not blind to the horrors of war. In the absence of solid information, the imagination often reaches for the worst. If the loved one does not know about PTSD, he or she can be scared and confused about why the Service Member has changed. They may even feel that they have done something wrong or that the traumatized individual is acting out of spite.

"How were things atypical when your husband got back from Iraq, as opposed to other deployments?"

"He was different, cold. At first, I thought he might be seeing someone else, but I heard from other military spouses that this had happened to them too. Some of their husbands were in all-male units, and I didn't think there could have been that many who turned gay during the deployment. Besides, it wasn't just the distance. Bill was different in so many ways. I knew the war had changed him."

"How so?"

"He wouldn't sleep, or if he did he would start screaming in the middle of the night. Because of that, I started not sleeping, either. I became irritable myself. When I snapped at him, he came back with a temper that was ten times worse than anything I had seen before. Then we both started distancing ourselves, avoiding the issue. He didn't trust me or anyone else, and I started not to feel safe around him."

Several studies have documented the cycle that Susan was describing, a pattern in which loved ones start to acquire the same difficulties as the individual who has PTSD. It is unclear if this is caused by vicarious trauma, or if, as Susan described it, cycles of sleeplessness, anger, mistrust, and avoidance feed on one another.

"You said that you didn't feel safe around him. Were you worried that he would actually hurt you or the children?"

"For the most part, no. At night, he would sometimes wake up swinging his fists. He even tried to strangle me once, but he would snap out of that quickly. Once I realized what was happening, and that he came out of it in a few seconds, I could deal with that. We kept separate beds. When he drank, though, that's the only time I worried about what he would do."

"And were you worried about your own behavior at all?" I asked. It is a difficult issue to broach when talking to a person you are trying to help, but violence can beget violence. In one study of Vietnam Veterans with PTSD, spouses reported committing more acts of family violence than the Veterans. It is unclear if this finding holds up across the board, but no matter what, it is always important to make sure that children are safe.

Luckily, Susan did not seem offended. "I know my temper has been up, too," she said. "I've been more hostile in general. I know I would never hit them, but I have said things to the kids that I know I shouldn't have."

When children are dealing with PTSD, it is important to create a safe place, a way for them to escape from the strange things Daddy or Mommy has been doing since getting back from war. We could talk about that at the end of the session, however. For now, I needed to create a safe place for Susan, let her know that she could talk about these things without being judged.

"Parenting is the toughest job in the world," I said. "All of us say things that we shouldn't from time to time. It's really good that you have recognized your own stress and the stress in the family. It can help you to plan to say the right thing next time."

"I don't know the right thing to say, not to the kids, and certainly not to Bill."

"Was the idea ever broached that there might be something clinically wrong with Bill?" I asked.

"He did go see a doctor once. They gave him pills, but they made our sex life even worse than it already was, so he stopped taking them."

Unfortunately, as Susan had described, medications that treat PTSD can sometimes have sexual side effects. The meds tend to inhibit drive more than they impair performance. In particular, they tend to delay orgasm, which is not always bad. However, even more so than when there is erectile difficulty, a spouse may perceive rejection if the patient stops initiating sex.

"Again, it is good that you recognized that it was the medication and not you," I said.

"I'm not so sure about that," Susan looked dejected. "He had already stopped touching me before he was taking the pills, and he didn't start up again much even after he stopped taking them."

"That doesn't mean that it was you," I explained. "Stress itself can decrease sex drive. Also, you mentioned that he was acting out violently at night. He may have been afraid to get too close to you. Drinking can cause sexual problems too. It is likely that he found you as attractive as ever, but it is easy to feel otherwise. Did you find that your image of yourself was suffering?"

"I'm a poster child for low self-esteem," she said. "I feel guilty about all of this: that I can't fix it, that I sometimes yell at him and the kids, that I might have sent him back to a place that could make him worse."

"First of all, you didn't send him there," I reminded her. "Second, we don't know if he is worse. What we do know for now is that you have gotten to the end of your rope yourself."

"I do feel that way," she said. "But I feel guilty about that too. He's the one who is in Iraq. How can I complain about my little suburban problems?"

"I'm not minimizing what your husband is going through, but the military does train its Service Members for deployment. There is no training for being a military spouse. We are seeing higher rates of depression, anxiety, and health issues in family members of those who deploy, especially if the Service Member is suffering from post traumatic stress. It definitely impacts you too."

Susan looked taken aback for a moment, and I realized that I had diagnosed her husband without actually meeting him. Although I strongly suspected that PTSD was the issue, I really didn't know, and neither did Susan.

"I don't know that your husband has post traumatic stress disorder," I backtracked, "but you are describing things that certainly make me suspicious. I'll give you some literature on the disorder, and we can talk about it if you like. If he does or he doesn't, you are still the person in this office, here and now. We need to pay attention to your well-being. If he does have PTSD, it is going to be difficult, and you are going to need to be as healthy as you can be to help him recover. No matter what, being a military spouse is tough."

Susan chewed on her lower lip. She took a long time before asking, "What if I'm not sure I want to help him anymore?"

"That's up to you," I said. "It is possible that the whole relationship is toxic, but it is also possible that you could help each other. A strong family is one of the best predictors of recovery for both partners. Sometimes even a dysfunctional family is better than no family at all. That may be less true for women than for men, however. You have to decide for yourself where the line is between helping and hurting. Certainly, if things have gotten to the point that you don't feel safe, the first thing you need to do is make sure that you have a way to get out if you need to. No matter what, the safety of you and your children has to come first. Also, it is possible that, even if you decide that you want to hold the family together, things could end in divorce. It takes two people to make a marriage work. If your husband is suffering from PTSD, it means that divorce is twice as likely to happen as it is for a military marriage where PTSD isn't involved. Hope for the best, but be prepared for the worst."

"I do want to stay, and I do want to help him. I don't know that I'm up to it, though. I don't think I can fix him."

"You definitely can't fix him," I said. "Only he can do that. But you can help, if he will let you. You can encourage him to get treatment. Gentle education from family members is often what brings Service Members into a psychiatrist's office. Also, family and friends can work together to do an intervention for alcohol problems. You can minimize risks by getting alcohol and firearms out of the home to begin with. Most important, you can keep yourself healthy. I'm going to ask you some more questions about clinical depression and anxiety. If they are positive, we might consider medications or therapy for you. No matter what, I recommend that you keep coming in to talk. Finally, I think you should get in touch with some support services to help both you and your children."

Susan looked a little overwhelmed by all that was being thrown at her. "Is this written down anywhere?" she asked.

"Lots of places and in lots of different ways. There is even information for kids. *Sesame Street* has a program for the younger ones. For those a little older, the Department of Defense published a comic book about PTSD. The Doonesbury comic strip also produced a series of books with characters who are Veterans. Each one shows how families and Service Members deal with combat, injury, PTSD, and even with traumatic brain injury. For adults, I usually recommend starting with the pamphlets that we have available at health clinics and Veterans centers. Internet searches aren't bad either, but as with everything on the Internet, you have to be careful about what a search engine produces. It's not a bad way to find support groups in your area.

"The Department of Defense came late to the idea that it was going to have to help military families, but the fact is that when a Service Member goes to Iraq or Afghanistan, the family goes to war as well. It is different than what the Service Member goes through, but that doesn't mean it is less serious. Luckily, the system is starting to catch up, and there are a lot of resources out there now for you, your children, and your husband."

"Do you really think he might come back OK, that we might be OK?"

"I do think it is possible," I said. "I've seen it happen."

# 16

# Virtual Reality Faces the Real Thing

THE virtual reality equipment in my office in Camp Fallujah gathered dust. By dust, I mean sand. The sand in Iraq is fine, and it settled as a brown film across anything not sealed airtight. When the sandstorms came through, the dust worked its way into even the deepest parts of the buildings and into the crevices of anything therein. The fine grains were gumming up the USB ports on my computers.

We had known the climate might eat the machines when I had borrowed the VR system from Mark Wiederhold before the deployment.

"You want to do the study out there?" he had asked.

"No, nothing formal. To be honest, I'm not even sure how, or even if, I'm actually going to use it. I don't have a protocol, a review board, or a specific plan. I just figure that since I'm going to be in the position of recommending to other doctors if they should take a machine into the field, I want the personal experience to back up what I say."

Mark had paused, probably realizing that not only was I asking him to send one of his expensive computer systems to be destroyed by the conditions of war but also for a project that could hurt his business if the results didn't turn out the way we hoped. Virtual reality was developing a good track record stateside. Military agencies were investing in system development, assuming that the same results could eventually be applied in the field, but so far that theory hadn't been put to the test.

"Do you honestly think it will help you with the troops?" he asked.

"I can't be sure, but given what I've seen so far, yeah, I think it will be useful."

"OK, then," he said. "We'll have one for you by the time you get on the plane."

True to his word, Mark had a machine ready for me when I started on my journey. So far, however, my prediction that it would be useful had yet to come true. It had been a royal pain in the butt to transport across the desert and now served as little more than a dust-covered decoration in the corner of my office in Camp Fallujah.

"I could get you compressed air to clean that out," said Major De-Santo, indicating the VR simulator, as he came in for our weekly visit.

"That might be useful." I motioned for him to sit down in the equally sand-coated chair across from me. "But I didn't think you were interested in treatments for PTSD?"

"I'm not," he said. "But anything that is an enemy to this sand is a friend to me." The major brushed himself off, adding another layer to the room. He had walked across camp to come to my office and was still coughing the stuff out. The dusty color muted the gray hue of his Air Force fatigues, making them seem more like the desert brown of the Marines.

Major DeSanto had started coming for appointments a few weeks ago, initially saying that he only wanted something to help him sleep. We had been practicing relaxation techniques using biofeedback. A small machine measured the major's heart rate and other aspects of his physiology. This let him know when the techniques were working. We also had talked about his life, which he always presented in vague terms. Sometimes I pushed the idea that it would be worth digging deeper.

"So, still nothing in particular that is bothering you this week? Nothing in your present, nothing in your past?" I asked.

The major paused. We had gone through this before—his classic symptoms of PTSD. He had nightmares about combat. He couldn't sleep. He didn't want to think or talk about anything to do with his first deployment. He avoided his friends, his family, thinking about the future. He had gone from being known as an officer who always kept his cool to a man feared by junior staff because he would fly into fits of rage at the drop of a hat.

When the major filled out our checklists of PTSD symptoms, no box was left unmarked. But, by themselves, checklists do not a diagnosis make. The major insisted that it was the stress of being in an administrative job that was getting to him. More important, from a diagnostic point of view, there wasn't any particular event, either in his past or present, that he identified as having started his symptoms.

"Let's say," Major DeSanto continued tentatively, "because I want to see if those machines actually start, that we did try them out. How would that work?"

It was my turn to pause. There is an expression: *When you have a shiny new hammer, everything looks like a nail.* I had dragged a high-tech hammer for PTSD halfway around the world. I wanted to make sure that I didn't let my enthusiasm for the technology pressure the major into a treatment that wasn't right for him. However, it seemed like he had the same symptoms that the virtual reality simulation helped improve in the States.

"Well," I explained. "There are two ways we use the technology to treat PTSD. In the first, we identify the original source of your trauma. We then would have you tell the story of what happened that day and use the virtual-reality simulator to illustrate the things you were talking about. In essence, we would have you take on both the memory of the trauma, and the sights and sounds that bother you, all within the same therapy session."

This first technique was what I had used in the United States with Corporal Spinoza and was still the method that I advocated the most.

Major DeSanto shook his head no. "I know you think I'm suppressing, or repressing, or whatever it is, Doc, but I'm telling you, there is no particular story to tell. I'm willing to admit I changed after my first deployment, but there wasn't anything that stood out. We got shelled a few times. Convoys got blown up. People died. I'm man enough to admit I was scared, but nothing was really worse than anything else."

I continued. "There is a second method. It starts off similarly to what we have been doing already with biofeedback. We teach techniques to help you recognize and tolerate anxiety. Then you use those techniques in the virtual reality to take on simulations of combat stresses. As you learn to overcome discomfort, we gradually increase the stress level in the simulator. We also monitor your physiology to make sure that you keep pushing yourself, but don't get overwhelmed. At first, you don't even have to talk much about your experiences, but as things progress, we see if the images trigger particular memories or help you learn more about what it is that causes your symptoms."

The major looked again at the dust-covered machines in the corner, eyeing them as one might a strange, but not necessarily unfriendly, animal in the room. "And in the long run, this might help my sleep? Help my nightmares?"

"In the States, it helped people with that type of thing, yes."

"OK. Let's do it."

The next session, Major DeSanto arrived with two cans of computer cleaner. We dusted off the machines, two computers that ran the simulator, a third laptop that recorded the biofeedback information, the physiology sensor, and the VR-headset. They all seemed in working order. I introduced the simulator to him much the same way as Dr. Spira had shown it to me years ago. Even when dealing with the cutting edge, things change slowly.

"What you will see is reflected on this computer here." I indicated the largest of the three notebook computers. Connected to it were headphones and a virtual reality headset. "This computer runs something that looks very much like a video game of Iraq."

I turned on the machine and showed him an image on the screen, a picture of an Iraqi street with a burned-out car sitting at the edge of the field of vision. "What is shown on this screen is the same thing you will see in the headsets," I continued. "As you move your head or body, the simulation will react as if you were moving in this virtual world."

"And you control the environment from the other computer. I get that," the major said. "But it doesn't look much like my office here."

I pushed a key on the controller computer, and the image shifted to a hospital. It looked like most medical facilities in the United States, except for the desert view through the windows and signs in Arabic. The simulated hospital was much larger and better appointed than our actual facility in Fallujah. Also there was no dust in the virtual reality. The major didn't seem to mind.

"I know it's an imperfect simulation," I explained. "We actually want it that way to begin with. The idea is to allow you to recognize what does bother you, and to slowly make it more realistic and more stressful, so that you learn to deal with those anxiety-provoking situations once you know what they are. In the first sessions, we will always agree ahead of time what you want to happen. As things progress, I may bring in some surprises, such as the sound of explosions. None of that will happen, however, until you are ready."

"And how will you know I'm ready?" The major looked anxious.

"The most important way is that you will tell me," I said. "But that is also where the third computer comes in. This machine will monitor your physiology. It is similar to the biofeedback device we have been using to help you relax and sleep. The main difference is that it provides much more detailed information, not just your heart rate but also your breathing, your body temperature, and how sweaty your palms are. The computer processes all this information to give me a readout about how stressed your body is. Instead of having you practice with a machine at home, like we did when we were using biofeedback for sleep, I will be the one monitoring your physiology while you are in the simulator. You don't really have to think about relaxing at all. Just do what comes naturally. If I see that you are very relaxed, then I will encourage you to take on greater challenges. If after a while, it looks like you are not able to calm down, or habituate, as we say, then we will try something easier the next time. Does that sound fair enough?"

Major DeSanto didn't answer, but put his hands out to take the headset. He placed it gingerly over his field of vision and adjusted the straps to tighten it on his clean-shaven head. I clicked a key on the controller computer and saw that we had him starting in a simulated base camp.

The major turned to his left and right, getting used to the way the system worked. As he turned his head to the right, I could see what was being projected into his goggles. A group of Service Members wandered across the sandy ground, while an American flag flapped above the simulated, walled compound. In the background was smoke, but it was unclear whether it came from a burn pit in the camp or from fires outside.

"How does that feel?" I asked. I had already observed that his heart rate and other physiological signs of anxiety had increased slightly. That surprised me, since the simulation was not too different from the environment he left to come to the hospital. I thought it might be the unfamiliar feel of the headset, but he gave me an answer I didn't expect.

"I know this is going to sound strange," he said. "But in some ways it feels more real than being here in Iraq now. It's like I can feel the weight of a flak jacket as soon as I start moving around here."

"And where does here look like?"

"More like Al Asad, where I was during my first deployment. Not so much like the camp here."

This came as another surprise. I had come through Al Asad on the convoy out to Fallujah. To me, it didn't look anything like the simulation on the screen. Al Asad was a massive base, with aircraft and runways. The simulation was of a small compound with tents. To me, it looked more like Camp Fallujah, where we were now.

Then it dawned on me. We didn't have that many tents left in Fallujah. Hard structures had replaced those a few years back. Really, the patchy nature of the video-game-like simulation didn't match either Al Asad or Fallujah. The simulation existed nowhere except in the mind of a programmer. I had seen a small camp and projected on it my memories of the world around us now. For the major, memories of Al Asad were stronger, so those thoughts had filled the gaps. Both of our imaginations were filling in, and for Major DeSanto, memory was powerful.

"OK, I think I'm ready to move on," the major said, bringing me back to the present. I advanced the simulator to the battlefield, and we continued our session.

Over the next several weeks, Major DeSanto came in regularly. In the simulation, we progressed from wandering inside the camp to exiting through the front gate to wandering in the nearby city and the tight spaces between Iraqi homes. Slowly, we introduced more stressful simulations, two medics working on a fallen American Service Member or the sound of gunfire coming steadily closer. The major adapted quickly, much more quickly, in fact, than patients with whom I had worked stateside.

Each time he had a session, Major DeSanto filled out a checklist of symptoms. I was pleased to see that issues were moving from the "severe" to the "mild" side of the sheet as we progressed. Things seemed to be going well. Then, about six sessions into treatment, something unusual happened.

"Holy crap!" the major jumped. "I thought you weren't going to throw in new sounds without telling me."

A resounding boom had shaken the office in the midst of our session. I felt my own pulse jump in synchrony with the changes the readout screen reflected for Major DeSanto. Ripples shook through the room and echoed in a cold cup of coffee on the edge of my desk. It wobbled and then fell, forming a kind of small, ceramic aftershock to the earlier explosion.

"That wasn't the simulator." I noticed, as if in slow motion, that both my voice and the major's were calmer than I would have expected in such a situation. "Take deep breaths. Then I'm going to ask you to take off the headset. We are going to move to the center of the building."

Moving to the center of the building was what Gunny Grant had told us to do the last time we came under rocket attack. I suddenly remembered that I had left my helmet in the other room.

Major DeSanto moved to comply, but before he could disentangle himself, another noise came blasting through the room. This time it was a voice on a loudspeaker.

"Controlled det! Controlled det! Remain at stations!" the voice announced.

"Crap, that was a big one," the major chuckled. His laughter was anxious, but in the way of someone who has been embarrassed at having jumped. His eyes darted to the mess on the floor. "Pity about your coffee. I thought they were supposed to warn us when they did that."

"They are supposed to." I laughed also and wiped up the spilled liquid. The major was referring to a controlled detonation, an explosion on base for a specific purpose. For example, if an enemy bomb is discovered, it may be brought back and blown up rather than taking the risk of trying to diffuse it in the field. Ordnance disposal teams are very good at what they do, so we were undoubtedly never in danger. However, sometimes they are in a rush and don't have time to let us know that they are about to shake the base. Also, this controlled detonation had been much more powerful than usual. It had felt very much like a real rocket attack.

I looked at the screen monitoring the major's physiology and noticed that his pulse was falling at about the same rate as I felt my own heart rate normalize.

"You did very well with that," I commented.

"You're right. I did." He seemed genuinely pleased. "You know, even when I knew they were coming, controlled dets have been making me jump out of my skin. Back in the States, a car backfiring would amp me up for days. That's the first time I've laughed about a loud noise since I got back from Iraq the first time."

"That certainly sounds like progress." I, too, was pleased.

"Funny thing is, I was afraid of just the simulated sound before. I'm not sure I would have let you set off an explosion in the virtual reality ten minutes ago."

"Now it doesn't seem like it would be so bad?"

"Naw, go ahead and do it." The major repositioned the virtual reality headgear.

Dutifully, I pushed the button that created a simulated IED explosion in the virtual world. A boom, nowhere near as loud as the one we had just heard, came out of the speakers and earphones.

"How did that feel?" I asked.

The major shrugged. "It still brings back memories," he said. "But I don't feel hyped up by it the way I used to. I feel like if it had been the real thing that I would have reacted appropriately."

Reacting appropriately was something for which Service Members here rapidly developed a knack. Sessions had occasionally been interrupted by the call for a mass casualty. This meant that US Service Members or our allies had been injured and would be rushed to the nearest military medical facility. All medical personnel, including me, had to stop whatever we were doing to attend to the trauma stations. The odds were low of being overwhelmed to the point that a psychiatrist would have to tend to a burn or blast victim, but we had to be prepared. In the States, a psychiatric patient in crisis would not have reacted well to this. The tragedy, and being abandoned in the middle of treatment, would have been too much. In Iraq, each time, no matter who was in session, he or she always took it with equanimity. In war, there are things that simply must be done.

"I think you are ready to move to a higher level," I said to Major DeSanto. I looked both at the monitor and at the major's eyes for signs of wavering, but there were none. His overcoming the controlled detonation had given us both confidence. We needed to take advantage of that. "This time through, I'm going to throw the kitchen sink at you in the simulator. I want you to walk out in the open, right down the middle of the street. I'm going to put you in a full-blown firefight. More important, I'm going to put you in a firefight that might look like something you actually witnessed during your first deployment. This time, I want you to not just tolerate the experience but also engage with it. I want you to tell me what the images remind you of, what actually happened."

The major nodded, showing the same resolve as when he had first put on the virtual reality headset. "We were about ten kilometers outside Bagdad," he said. "The main road was closed because another convoy had broken down a few hours earlier. The alternate was mostly good, except for one place where we had to go through a tight spot between houses."

In the simulator, I teleported him to a place that was the closest approximation I could guess of what he was describing. "Yeah, it was like this," the major continued. "Except that we were driving rather than on foot, and there were more people around." I didn't have anything to match those changes in the simulator, so I let him continue in the imperfect approximation.

"You are doing great," I said. The major's heart rate and breathing had quickened, but it was nothing that looked like panic.

"The buildings were close, and we couldn't see who was in the windows. It was the perfect spot for an ambush. Sure enough, as we are halfway down, a sniper starts popping off rounds."

Pop. Pop. Pop. From the controller computer, I called up the sounds of an AK-47 firing.

Digital graphs on the physiology computer told me that the major's hands were sweating, but again, still no signs of panic. "How did you feel at the time?' I asked.

"Scared, of course, and a little confused. I wouldn't call it a full-blown firefight, but I didn't think that as an Air Force officer I was going to be involved in ground combat."

"You are still doing great," I said. "What happened next?"

"We fired a few rounds back at the rooftops, but the CO told us to hold off from using the larger, vehicle-mounted weapons. We couldn't see where the firing was coming from, and we didn't want to take out buildings full of civilians. Mostly, we let off smoke so the sniper couldn't get a clear shot. We gunned the engines to push on through. I always felt bad knowing that we had left the sniper alive to open up on other Americans."

"And you never talked to anyone about this?" I asked.

"I never thought it was that important," he explained. "As I said, it wasn't much of a firefight, and we did let the bad guy get away."

"But there were bullets flying by your head?"

"Maybe it did keep me up at night for a while. I guess I'm getting better about it now."

And he did get better. We replayed that scenario several times during that session, and again the following week. Each time, the quickening of his pulse became less. After a while, the major told me he was sleeping better and that he really did need to get back to work.

"I'll tell people that this helped me, though," the Major said in our last session, while explaining that he didn't think he would be back.

Apparently, he did tell others, because soon I had about half a dozen patients with PTSD who were coming in for treatment. It still accounted for a relatively small percentage of my practice in Fallujah, but dust stopped accumulating on my virtual reality machines.

Meanwhile, Dr. Barnum's campaign to embed herself with the regular Marine units was paying off. She also had accumulated a small cadre of patients who had PTSD from previous deployments.

"Are you noticing that clients with PTSD here seem to get better faster than when we treat them in the States?" she asked one morning, as we both filled our mugs with coffee outside our side-by-side offices.

"Definitely," I said. "I'm using mostly the virtual reality treatment. I'm not sure if it is because of that technique or if it has more to do with the fact that people are also taking on the real thing."

"Or, since most of what we see is preexisting, it could mean that the Service Members who come out here despite their PTSD are particularly motivated," Dr. Barnum postulated. "Also, they had to slip past the screening system, which means that a lot of them never told anyone about their issues before. If you have been bottling something up for years, any chance to open up about it is going to seam cathartic."

I reflected on this, but my experience said that wasn't all there was to it. "I have a patient who was a reservist," I explained. "He went back to civilian life between deployments. He was in regular talk therapy for a couple of years. It didn't make him better. He came out here, thinking that he could fix things this time around, but after two months back in Iraq, his symptoms were still the same. Just a few sessions here, and his PTSD improved dramatically. I think there is something in the idea that taking on your past, both in thought and in deed, is essential to cure."

Dr. Barnum answered, "That's kind of how traditional prolonged exposure therapy works for civilian trauma. Someone who had been in a car accident would both have to talk about the accident and get back in cars."

"You are using traditional prolonged exposure therapy, right?"

"For the most part. Like everything else out here, we have to adapt techniques to the environment."

"Still, we should compare notes when we finish up here, see which technique worked best."

She agreed and went back to her morning coffee. I wondered if I might be getting overconfident about treatment in theater. I had a patient who came in with only a week left before heading home. I tried to treat him anyway. I hadn't cured him, but then again, he hadn't gotten worse either. But what if traditional treatment was better? Or, worse, what if virtual reality was desensitizing patients too quickly? What if they lost their edge?

When HM2 Jimenez came in to his next session, I decided to ask him about this. HM2 stands for hospital man second class. Jimenez was a corpsman, a Navy medic, who had been through two previous tours in Iraq and Afghanistan. He had seen things that would have overwhelmed the most experienced trauma surgeons. Corpsmen are the Navy and Marine Corps' "first line of defense" for any medical problems, and I knew that even while he was in treatment, he was out in the field treating medical trauma every day.

"How have your responses to emergencies changed during treatment?" I asked, as we debriefed from his last virtual reality session. He had been telling me about a mass casualty during his first deployment. As he told this story over and over while the virtual reality simulated violence, he had come to terms with his past, accepted that there was no way that he could have saved everyone, that it was not his fault. But did that make him numb?

"No, not numb," he said. "I'm more calm, more in the moment."

"Is that ever a bad thing? Is it hard now that you aren't cutting yourself off from your emotions?"

"It *is* hard," he explained. "But I think it is better to be in touch with what you feel. The other day, we came across an Iraqi bus that had driven into a ditch. They don't use seatbelts much here. The scene was pretty gory. Gas was everywhere, and a match could have made it into one big crematorium. Before I was in treatment, I would have asked to sit this one out. I would have thought I couldn't handle it. What if I ended up having flashbacks right there in the field? But now I knew that wouldn't happen. We had gone through worse in the simulator, and I did fine. I was aware that I was scared, but that that was OK."

I asked, "You weren't retraumatized?"

"I hadn't really thought about it," he said. "I guess it could have been horrific, but it wasn't. It was just part of my job. It was what I had to do."

Having a job to accomplish seemed a common theme among people who recovered while in Iraq. Friedrich Nietzsche said that "he who has a why to life, can bear almost any how." Perhaps people didn't need to go back to war to face their demons, but maybe they did have to find something that was worth fighting for.

By the time I left Iraq, I still wasn't sure whether the virtual reality was the factor that helped people. It could have been that seeing them perform well in the simulator gave me the confidence to send them back to their jobs. Maybe it was the job itself, the purpose that allowed them to recover. What was clear, however, is that even in the midst of the greatest challenges, people can persevere. Service Members in Iraq did take on the simulator. They also took on real life, and, often, they won.

# 17

# Different Roads Home

YOU can't go home again." That's what Thomas Wolfe said, but we knew better. It was August in Iraq, and we were scheduled to return to the United States in September. Home was a palpable prize, a glimmering oasis in the blistering heat of the Iraqi summer.

"There is nothing quite like the feeling when the wheels of the plane touch down on American soil," explained Gunnery Sergeant Grant, a three-time veteran of deployments to Iraq. "It's Christmas, the Fourth of July, and the birth of your first child all rolled into one. But we have work to do before we get going. The enemy likes to test us in the transitions, so stay sharp."

Statistically, the beginning and end of deployments are the most dangerous. As Gunny said, the enemy likes to test us. The new troops coming in are green, and the old ones going out have their minds on other things. It's the perfect time for an attack. Knowing this, our minds were still on other things.

"There is a customer for you at Baharia," HM2 Delphin explained, having returned from a briefing in the command conference room. "They have a suicidal Marine over there but are having problems calming him down enough to transport him to us."

"We could go to him, I suppose," I said. Baharia was the next base over from Camp Fallujah. It had once been a Bathist resort frequented by Qusay and Uday Hussein before the 82nd Airborne took it over, destroying most of the recreational buildings in the process. Baharia was nicknamed "Dreamland" because of a documentary called *Occupation Dreamland* about the 82nd's exploits in Iraq. It held a certain mystique in military circles.

Even as the words left my mouth, I realized my suggestion was based more on curiosity than on the urgency of the medical situation. I was getting ready to leave Iraq, and I had seen almost nothing of the country. The majority of my deployment had been spent within the seven-mile perimeter of Camp Fallujah. My only forays out had been done either by helicopter or within the windowless canvas of seven-ton trucks. A trip to Baharia would mean commandeering an SUV or a Humvee, a window seat. It would mean a chance to actually see the world outside.

"I don't think that's the best idea, Sir," said Petty Officer Delphin. "I'm sure the Marines will figure this out and get the patient to us within an hour or so."

Delphin was both correct and properly cautious. He had a Purple Heart from having been hit by an IED during his last deployment. Baharia was only a five-minute drive from our base and along a well-guarded road, but why should we take chances?

The words had been spoken, however, and others picked up on the idea.

"I can get you a vehicle," chimed in Commander Becerra. "We can take along Rodney and Norm for security."

Commander Becerra was a neurologist officially stationed with headquarters in an administrative role but spent most of his time with us at the hospital. Rodney and Norm were our flight nurse and physician assistant, respectively. There was some sense in their playing a security role. Norm was a former Navy SEAL, and Rodney was large enough that he would have made an intimidating bodyguard if his calling were to violence rather than to healing. We all knew, however, that this was, again, an excuse. If we had really wanted security guards, there were Marines with that job description.

Commander Becerra, Norm, Rodney, and I were one another's closest friends on base. The shared toil and dormlike living conditions had

formed us into a clique, the likes of which I had not been a part since
college. Although we were all grown men, we were again acting like
college students on a fraternity outing. Commander Becerra grabbed
the keys to one of the hospital's SUVs and signed us out as going to
Baharia. Captain Cogar, the hospital CO and the one person in the
medical facility who outranked Commander Becerra, was conveniently
away when he did so. A Navy commander is the equivalent rank to a
Marine lieutenant colonel, so no one else was going to challenge his
request. The rest of us grabbed our helmets and firearms and piled into
the vehicle.

The short trip between Camp Fallujah and Baharia was uneventful.
What passed for roads was heavily pot-holed dirt. Most of the traffic we
saw was other military vehicles. Ours was the only car that wasn't armored, but with the US and Iraqi armies around us on the road, we never
felt unsafe. Rodney photographed the sights through the passenger-side
window. We slowed for better shots when we passed the occasional
bombed-out building and a huge junkyard of twisted, military-looking
metal, presumably the remains of what had once been Saddam Hussein's
army. Soon we approached the Iraqi and American flags of the Camp
Baharia entry checkpoint.

We slowed and weaved around the concrete barriers to approach the
guards at the gate.

"Welcome to Camp Baharia, gentlemen." The guard waved us forward after checking our identifications. "Please return your weapons to
condition four as you pass onto base."

"Oh, yes, of course," I stammered, as our vehicle moved forward.
When off base we were supposed to put weapons in condition one,
meaning that a round is chambered and the gun is ready to fire. I had
forgotten to do so and had left my sidearm in condition four, meaning
unloaded, the whole time. Flustered by my oversight, I neglected to ask
the guard the way to the medical facility.

"The base isn't that big," reassured Norm reassured. "I'm sure we'll
find it."

As we circled the wrong way around the man-made lake that defined
the center of Baharia, a far longer drive than our voyage between bases,
the call came in that the patient I was there to see had already left. He
was on his way to my office in Camp Fallujah.

"Well, we better get back then," said Commander Becerra, and we again drove the short, uneventful distance between Camp Baharia and Camp Fallujah.

The CO was waiting for us when we got back.

"You are all adults, so I'm not going to lecture you on how stupid that was," said Captain Cogar. "But you should know that they dug enemy mines out of that road last week. Just because it's been relatively quiet here on base doesn't mean that there isn't still a war on. Next time, at least get the Marines to drive you over in an armored vehicle."

We all do dumb things from time to time. Our car had been filled with people with a half-dozen graduate degrees and more than sixty years of military experience. Yet we had let the excitement of going home and the need for last-minute adventure overwhelm our better judgments. All along that trip, we had made bad decisions and made rookie mistakes. With safety being so close at hand, it was easy to see how, if things had gone otherwise, we could have spent a lifetime beating ourselves up for our decision. Also, although our act of foolishness was to take unneeded risks, sometimes the actions go the other way. In combat, the inappropriate choice to be too conservative or timid can cause as many casualties as the decision that throws caution to the wind.

"In the final days, the tragedies start to seem heavier," Captain Cogar later said, explaining how he had worried. "We see these kids come through the hospital now, and you have to think, if they could have stayed safe for a few days longer."

We heard about many of these closing-day tragedies. Our particular hospital didn't get overwhelmed with the wounded, but we knew something had gone wrong when all communications to the United States would be suddenly cut off. It usually meant that a Service Member had been killed or injured. The communications freeze was in place so that the news came to the family through official channels rather than via the rumor mill. But ending communications to the States didn't cut off the rumors on base.

"I heard an insurgent jumped the wire last night," someone said. "Opened fire with a revolver into the motor pool tents. He got away too. How crazy is that. Someone with a revolver jumps into a base filled with ten thousand armed Soldiers and Marines, and he gets away."

"I heard they tried to poison our water supply. It wasn't very effective, but that's why our water was out for three days last week."

"Someone told me that they are shutting this base down, that we will be turning it over to the Iraqis when we leave."

"I heard that some of us are going to have to stay on when they shut it down, that we are going to be assigned to the medical unit at Tikrit. That will extend us by another three months."

The last rumor was the most destructive. When I came to Iraq, the constant back and forth about if and when I was leaving had been incredibly stressful. I could only imagine how much worse it would be if the dreamed-of date to return home kept retreating into the future. The suicidal Marine about whom we had been called turned out to have experience with this.

"On my last deployment, we were extended," he explained. "We had already done our time. We were ready for that, but it is so much worse when you aren't prepared. Each time we got into a firefight, it was another reminder that we weren't supposed to be here, that we were supposed to be home safe with our families by now. I don't think I can take that again."

As it turned out, his unit was really leaving the next day. We sent him home, and he did fine. He wasn't totally off about the rumors of extension, however. The following day, Captain Cogar was asked if he would be willing to take new orders to Afghanistan.

"It's for the position of medical director for the entire theater of operations. They are offering it as an opportunity," he explained. "They haven't said anything directly, but the implication is that if I do this, I might have a shot at making admiral."

The move from captain to admiral in the Navy, equivalent to the promotion from colonel to general in other branches, is exceedingly rare for a medical officer. It is the ultimate pinnacle of a military career.

"It has to be tempting," I said.

"A bit. But in the end, my kids are more important," Captain Cogar explained. "My son is already mad at me for being gone this long. It's time to come home."

Promotion isn't the only temptation to stay in theater. At every rank level, there are financial incentives, combat pay, and tax breaks to stay on deployment. There is also the simple sense of purpose. Many Service Members describe that, no matter the stresses of deployment, combat means that one's job is boiled down to its essence. Sometimes, you want to finish what you started.

For the most part, the choice to extend a deployment is not one the military lets you take. Modern armies have studied burnout and are well aware that after a certain point troops become less effective. They need to go home. For this reason, the US Marine Corps tries to keep deployment lengths to seven months, the Army to twelve months. This may seem short to students of history who remember that troops in World War II and other conflicts were away for years at a time. Since Vietnam, however, improved intelligence and mobility mean that the typical Service Member is moved into combat faster and more often than their historical predecessors and thus burn out faster.

The necessities of war, and the realities of an all-volunteer force, mean that those ideal limits are pushed. Reservists and those in highly specialized jobs often extend well beyond the ideal deployment time. The Army occasionally has had to increase its deployments to eighteen months or longer. Even in the best of times, some people are going to have to stay longer than they should.

"At least I had the choice about Afghanistan," Captain Cogar continued. "Some of us are going to be extended in Iraq. They will be shutting down Camp Fallujah, so we need to be prepared to move or take on new assignments as they come up."

Breaking up a unit can be a particularly difficult aspect of the redeployment home. No matter the hardship, a unit builds its own support system. Everyone knows how everyone else works. Everyone is his brother's keeper. Even if you are one of the lucky ones and get sent home on schedule, knowing that you are leaving your fellow Service Members behind is never easy.

The following weeks marked a period of breaking down structures and throwing things away. The official word was that the camp, when turned back over to the Iraqis, would be in the same condition as when we took it over. All signs of things American had to be expunged. We lined up to empty sandbags and to break bookcases. In a sense, this seemed incredibly wasteful. Wasn't a sandbag a sandbag, no matter who filled it?

At least the manual labor of breaking down the base gave us a chance to all work together. We lined up, officer and enlisted, doctors, nurses, and lab techs, all to do the honest labor of lifting and using our hands. The physical strain was cleansing.

"Careful for scorpions or spiders," our team's entomologist warned as we started off. "They like to hide in the dry wood."

We didn't need the warning. We had seen the effect of Iraq's insects first hand, as such injuries had come through the ER in previous months. Even while carefully checking for the small, deadly creatures, it was pleasant to think that in a few short weeks we would be returning to a place where bee stings were about the worst thing that one might expect from a bug.

We started the work early in the morning, while the temperatures in the shade hovered below the one-hundred-degree mark. By 10 a.m., the needle was climbing back into triple digits, and we decided to call it quits and return to clinical work for the day. We were dirty and hot but not unhappy.

"Look, the psychiatrist's shirt has a smile on it," laughed Dr. Jerome, one of our team's two dentists. He ran to grab his camera and showed me the image.

Sure enough, the sweat and grime on my shirt had formed into what appeared to be two eyes and a large grin. The garment was probably ruined, but it had ended its usefulness in a way that caused happiness and that was about the best that could be hoped for from an olive-drab t-shirt.

The t-shirt was thrown away, as were many other items from my room. During my deployment, I had collected a small hoard of knickknacks and keepsakes sent from home. Their value diminished immensely with the thought that whatever was retained would have to be carried on my back. There were a few items, a tape recording from my wife, a few books, that I wanted to keep but not carry. Luckily, the Marines had set up a postal annex from which packages could be sent back to the United States.

"I won't miss this heat," Rodney said, as we waited together in the line at the post office tent. We had already gone through about a liter of water each in the fifteen minutes we had been waiting in the sun. Rodney grabbed a thermometer that was sitting in its usual place in the tent and brought it out with us into the sun. It soon topped out at its maximum, 140 degrees Fahrenheit. We snapped pictures to send home later, hoping the heat wouldn't ruin the film before we had a chance to show them off.

"It's hard to believe we were lifting rocks at this temperature this morning," I said. "At home I give up on yard work if it gets to eighty-five."

Rodney agreed, the sweat pouring off his forehead. "I'll certainly never take air-conditioning for granted again."

I felt as if I'd never take things for granted: cool air, clean clothes, the safety of knowing that rocket shells are unlikely to drop on you as you sleep. Most important was the friendship of someone who will stand and take pictures with you in the insanity of the Middle Eastern sun.

Gunnery Sergeant Grant had talked about how arriving home felt like Christmas Day. To some extent, I already felt like I was in that season. I was counting my blessings and thinking I might go home changed for the good. Six months with the Marines had left me ten pounds lighter and probably in the best shape of my life. I had started on this book and finished writing several scientific papers that I had put off for years. I realized that the junk I had packed and accumulated on the trip was just that, junk. I needed very little to be happy. No matter what, I had it much better than the people who had to live their whole lives in a war zone. Even though I knew that the trip home would probably be the most physically dangerous part of the deployment, I wasn't afraid. I knew that I could trust the men and women with whom I served and that they would do their best to protect me. If by some fluke, they failed, I knew that I had led a blessed life, and that if I died I would not have been cheated by life.

The idea that difficult circumstances can lead to growth as well as disorder is not new. Nietzsche famously said "that which does not destroy us makes us stronger." In recent years, academics had taken to calling this "post traumatic growth." Of course, I realized that my own experiences had not been that traumatic. We did have some stress. I would later learn that at least one member of our medical company had felt traumatized and developed PTSD from dealing with the attacks and the medical casualties that came through our facility. But this was still within the range of expectation and interpretation. What about the individuals who were shot or lost a close friend? Was it possible that people who went through those experiences also felt that they would go home stronger?

I decided to ask about people who had gone through the worst and yet come out resilient. A number of names were volunteered. For example, there was a Marine in camp who had lost a leg in battle and yet was redeployed to Fallujah. He was out running on his prosthetic leg every day. The name that came up most often, however, was Colonel George Bristol, the commander of First Marine Expeditionary Force Headquarters Group.

It is natural that troops will look up to their commanding officer, but as I asked around, it became clear why Colonel Bristol was so admired. He had started as an enlisted Marine and worked his way up, largely by being the toughest guy in the room. And those rooms were filled with very tough guys. The colonel had been in infantry, reconnaissance, and, before fighting in the battle of Fallujah in 2004, had already been in Special Operations billets in areas that included Somalia, Bosnia, Central America, and the Far East. The rumor was that he worked for the CIA as well as the Marines, but one learned not to ask too many questions about that kind of thing. In the words of one Marine, however, he was who "you go to when you absolutely, positively have to kill someone tonight."

But Bristol's fame wasn't really about his personal fighting skills, although those were certainly formidable. The colonel had been instrumental in developing martial arts training for the Marines, and with this the idea that a code of ethics must be incorporated into Warrior training. Bristol was not the lone assassin of a movie stereotype but a commanding officer who cared for and mentored his troops.

He still presented an imposing figure when I came into his office and told him I wanted to ask him some questions about transitioning home. The colonel was a big man, by any standard, with a shaved head and a nose that looked as if it had been broken and reset many times. He extended a large, meaty hand but did not smile as I sat down in his office.

"So they told me the shrink wanted to ask me questions. I guess I should have expected that." The voice was gravelly and harsh, but it was clear that the statement was made with dry humor, not malice.

"Yes, Sir. I appreciate your time. As you know, our medical section is about to head home, and I wanted to talk to someone who had made the trip before and done it well."

"It's not easy going home," Bristol said gravely. "Sometimes it's even harder than going to war."

The colonel was generous with his time and with his views on returning home, but neither he nor I could, in the end, figure out what it was that made transition easy or hard.

"You are going to get cruel comments, stupid questions," Bristol said. "You have to be prepared for it. I've come to realize that when talking to people who have never been to war, they don't have the privilege of my pain."

Interestingly, at least one study suggested that Colonel Bristol had put his finger on it when he suggested that pain allowed him to become the man that he was. In Veterans of Iraq and Afghanistan, those with the most severe symptoms of post traumatic stress disorder were also the individuals who experienced the greatest positive changes. Other factors were important too, however, including unit support, and the sheer effort an individual put out. "The world breaks everyone," Ernest Hemingway wrote, "and afterward many are strong in the broken places."

I wondered if I would be able to show anything like the resilience of Colonel Bristol. Ironically, as the camp's mental health officer, I was the one briefing Service Members to remind them that the transition home might be harder than expected. As our trip to Baharia had shown, however, knowing something and having the wisdom to put it into practice are not the same thing.

No matter the dumb things I might do, I realized that I was lucky. I had both a relatively low-trauma deployment and good support waiting for me when I got home. Some of my patients were not so fortunate on either account. I was concerned about how they might do after the trip back.

Many Service Members with whom I had worked in Iraq had serious issues awaiting them at home—unfaithful spouses, financial burdens, a lifetime of abuse that would linger in their minds regardless of what country they found themselves in. Like me, a few were going back with the expectation that they would need to start looking for civilian employment as soon as they returned. As a psychiatrist, I knew there would be a job for me, somewhere. It was a scarier prospect for a Service Member whose main job proficiencies had been shooting straight and defusing bombs. Those skills translated into some security positions, but a history of psychiatric symptoms often scared off employers in the police and security fields.

"Are you ready for the trip home?" I asked each patient as we closed our final sessions together. Depending on the individual, this could mean: "Have you packed your medications?" "Do you know how to find a therapist stateside?" "Are you OK that we two, having shared together the most intimate stories of your life, will likely never speak again?"

Leaving a therapist can be a difficult experience, even when you aren't traveling across a battlefield and between civilizations to do so. Perhaps the trip home would finally provide relief for some war-weary Service Members, but I worried about the patients who had gotten better here. Would those who had been treated with virtual reality stay "cured"? Would nightmares and anger, which had vanished in the simulator, return when machine and desert were left behind? Would the ghosts of war remain locked in the machine, or would new demons form that were harder to control in the real world than in virtual reality?

I made a few calls to the States. Some of my patients had gone home ahead of us, and a few had left their phone numbers. "Are you doing OK?" I asked.

"Yes," was the invariable answer, although some admitted that they were going to continue in therapy for a while "to make sure." What did that mean? When it came to leaving this place behind, how could you ever be sure you were done with it?

Soon our replacements arrived, although without the midnight fanfare we were given when we had appeared in Camp Fallujah. Before the arrival of this new medical team, there had been confusion about whether we would be replaced at all. With the closing of the base, we thought medical care would be turned over to one of the larger facilities in the province. When the new group of doctors and nurses hopped off the truck outside our small hospital, it came as a surprise to all of us.

"I thought we were checking in to Baharia," said Dr. Johnson as I helped her carry her sea bags back to the medical quarters.

"There is only one mental health provider?" I asked. "Are you replacing both Dr. Barnum and me? The troop levels are going to be cut back, but, still, that would be a tough workload."

"Dr. Barnum has been given orders to extend," it was explained. "The regimental combat team didn't want to give her up."

I was going home. Dr. Barnum was not. In fact, the entire medical unit was going to be split up for our convoy home. Plans that Chief Perez had made for a barbecue together when we arrived in the United States would have to be changed. Some of the medical team would probably not even see one another again stateside, as those who lived on the East Coast divided from those returning to California.

"Are you OK?" I asked Dr. Barnum, a question I found myself repeating a lot lately.

"It's frustrating," she said. "I volunteered for the traveling shrink job knowing it might be the tougher choice, but it was what I wanted to do. Now it feels like I'm being punished for that. It's Ramadan in a few days anyway. The convoys are going to stop, so I'm not even going to be doing my job for the next month. But, yeah, I think I'm OK. Have a good trip home."

The convoy out of Camp Fallujah was as chaotic as the one on the way in. Crammed sardine-like into the back of the seven-ton truck, I was lucky enough to be near a small crack in the canvas that allowed a view of the passing world. Flickering images of the city and the countryside appeared in that hole as we drove through the dust of the desert. Often the trucks would stand still, stalled for unknown reasons. We mumbled complaints up and down the line of crammed-in bodies, coughing sand out of our lungs, and wondering how many hours more had been put between us and home. The flack and Kevlar protection grew heavier and pressed into my skin as we waited. My back ached from the weight, and I wondered how the troops who did this daily ever got home with spines intact. The flickering lights outside the truck eventually grew brighter, a sign that we were near the air base, perhaps? After several waves of false hope came the order to disembark.

We stepped out into the Al Asad Airbase and dragged our packs to the visitor tents to sleep, which we did hard and deeply. The next few days were spent waiting for the news of a plane to Kuwait. Other medical units, some with familiar faces, also passed through. We traded gossip and news of what to expect at the next stage. Some said we needed to be prepared to wait for weeks in Kuwait, in case they wanted to turn us around. It was probably best not to tell your family exactly when to expect you home. False hope and all.

Al Asad was better appointed than Camp Fallujah. The chow hall had better food, and the exchange sold souvenirs. I bought some old Iraqi money, with pictures of Saddam Hussein on the brightly colored paper, and a bottle of perfume for my wife. The perfume was dressed up in a Arabic-looking bottle, but I suspected it was a knockoff of an American brand. Someone told me they were all made in China anyway. I also got a not-surprisingly good deal on a leather coat. Such items weren't exactly selling well in what an accurate thermometer in the sun now identified as 156-degree heat. With my purchases, I realized that I was already abandoning my resolution to live a less materialistic life. But, hey, after months away from it, was there anything wrong with retail therapy?

Despite the new opportunities for food and shopping, the days seemed longer here, partly due to the waiting but also because I was idle. Waiting is harder when you have nothing to do. I wandered over to the mental health clinic to see what was going on.

"So what did you do with the virtual reality simulator when you left?" the psych tech there asked. I had previously told him about the equipment when we ran into each other in Baghdad a few months back.

"I left it behind," I said. "The Wiederholds want it to get more use, and I'm not carrying that thing twice. I showed Dr. Johnston how it works. Hopefully, someone will get some use out of it before the sandstorms destroy the electronics."

The C-150 plane out of Al Asad was bumpy but considerably more comfortable than the truck convoy. I remembered Gunny Grant's words about the feeling of wheels touching down on American soil, but I was happy enough when we lifted off from Iraq. I looked down on the vast

swath of desert that supposedly once contained the Garden of Eden and
counted my lucky stars that I was leaving in one piece.

"Kuwait is one ugly place," one Marine on the C-150 announced as
we disembarked.

"Not a terribly generous thing to say about our host country," I said,
"but from what I can see of it, I would have to agree."

"In Iraq, I get it," the Marine said. "The people can't leave, but the
Kuwaitis are rich. Why do they stay? None of it makes sense to me."

Again, I had to agree. It all seemed surreal, the countryside and the
military posture like Iraq, but the reality so very different. After dropping my pack at the transitional tent, I wandered around and settled into
the new country. After a few days, it seemed close enough to home that
I decided to send an e-mail announcing my impending return:

> I have made it out of Iraq, and am now in Kuwait. Kuwait is re-
> markably similar to Iraq in many aspects—hot, dusty, and free of
> anything green except the Jello. It is so similar, in fact, that the
> Iraqis appear to have confused it for their 19th province and started
> a bit of a mess back in the early '90s. Kuwait does have one, pro-
> found advantage over Iraq, however, in that no one here is trying
> to kill us. Well, no one except perhaps the taxi drivers. Wow, the
> driving here is bad. Technically, we are still in a combat zone (for
> tax code purposes anyway), but they took away all of our ammuni-
> tion, we packed our Kevlar away, and there are bus trips available
> to the mall. I know I have said the mall can sometimes seem like a
> combat zone, but this is getting silly. Anyway, it is one more step
> back toward the US of A, where I am sure that I will feel absolutely
> freezing at 80 degrees. Luckily, they are trying to acclimatize us
> early by keeping the air conditioner in our tent set at temperatures
> that make me suspect that it also doubles as a meat locker. Now
> that I think about it, that would also explain the smell, but, then
> again, that could also just be Marines. As they say, however, there
> is nothing bad about the trip home. This is still true, and I can't
> wait to be back. All the best, and hope to see you soon.

The next step home was Germany, a town called Landstuhl in the
southwest where the United States had set up a huge air base and medical

center. The gate attendants were polite in the usual German way and were also kind enough not to cringe at the odor as we disembarked. In Kuwait, before boarding the C-130, we had to stand out in the sun for two hours to go through a search to make sure that we were not smuggling antiquities or hand grenades out of the country. A river had skirted the sidewalk, and we were all aware that the source was not the Tigris and Euphrates but our own sweat. Hours more in the plane had not improved our hygiene.

The stay in Germany was brief, not long enough for a shower or even an escape to get a beer in a country in which it was now legal to drink. But there was something glorious in the small outdoor courtyard of the airport waiting area.

"Green grass!" someone exclaimed, as many in the group bent to run their hands through the dewy blades.

Here the small things were still valued, but most of the passengers were holding on for the promise of the next stop. We would have an hour in Ireland, and there, it was promised, would at last be beer.

I found myself abstaining in the land of Guinness, not because I didn't have a fondness for Irish beer, but because I felt I had to try to be something of an example. Stateside, alcohol problems were among the most common issues I saw in returning Service Members. Besides, I was already drunk on the idea of the next touchdown. That would finally be in the United States, with all the promises of a Christmas and Fourth of July landing.

The touchdown didn't feel special, but the people in Maine were particularly kind. Our plane landed in the wee hours of the morning, yet dozens of volunteers were out to greet us. The same people who had been there to wish us well as we left were also welcoming us home. Like the Germans, they politely ignored our smell. More so, they moved to hug us. They gave us cookies and phone cards to call our families. They called us heroes.

To be honest, the arrival felt awkward. The cookies were nice, but I knew I hadn't done anything particularly heroic in Iraq. This wasn't the volunteers' fault. There certainly were heroes getting off the plane with me, and the volunteers were far too nice to pick and choose whom to hug. Also, I didn't really need the phone card. I made a good living and could pay for the call to my wife myself. I was tired, and after weeks of traveling, the cost of having to engage in conversation with strangers at 2 a.m. seemed far greater than the value of the food or the free phone calls.

At the same time, as I felt strange about the greeting, I somehow knew that it would have been worse if the volunteers hadn't been there. I would have felt neglected. It was a weird, catch-22 situation, and one that, for the time being, I was too tired to think about.

Two more plane stops and then a bus, and we were finally back at Camp Pendleton, about an hour north of San Diego. It was twelve hours after our scheduled arrival time. The banners and flyers that had been hung were unreadable in the night. The food that had been prepared had been eaten hours ago, and the friends and family members that were waiting looked almost as tired as we did.

"Just go home," the officer in charge announced. "It's late, and we can muster and debrief in the morning. We'll leave your packs on the trucks until then. Anyone who needs a place to stay tonight, come with me. We'll take the bus on over to the barracks."

I didn't need a place to stay. I was home or at least an hour's car ride from home. Where was my wife, Lizzie? I had disconnected my cell phone while I was on deployment and had to find someone with a key to an office so I could find a landline.

Lizzie was in tears when I reached her. She was lost. She couldn't find her way around the base in the dark, and because she was crying, it was that much harder to communicate the directions. Could I drive when she got there? It was all too much.

I struggled with the mirrors on the car. Lizzie had made a reasonable request. At home, I had always been the one to do the driving. She did other chores that I liked far less. Driving on longer trips was my job. I just didn't expect to pick it back up so quickly when I returned.

The next day, I checked back in at Pendleton, unpacked, and tried to reach the members of my unit who had come back to Southern California. Chief's welcome back barbecue had fallen through, so I decided to hold one of my own. It would have to wait a week or so. Some members made it back a few days before me. Others still hadn't gotten in. That didn't include Dr. Barnum, who wouldn't return for another three months.

"Chicken, hamburgers, or ribs?" I said, standing at the grill at the quintessentially American backyard activity.

The barbecue was nice. Many friends attended, and it was good to get into my pool. We had bought the house just before I left for Iraq, and I never had the chance to swim there before now. I found myself annoyed with small things though. The fruit trees that I had planted around the outside of the yard had all died. Lizzie hadn't known how to work the sprinkler system. Other members of my unit noted similar complaints. The frustrations of everyday life were already settling in.

"People keep thanking me for my service," noted one of the corpsman, "but I'm being fined by a traffic court for missing a hearing yesterday from a ticket I got before we deployed. I had seven months of mail piled up when I got home. I'm sorry the hearing notice didn't pop right to the top when I walked through the door."

That complaint was minor compared with many others—house foreclosures, loss of child custody, marital infidelity, all of which seemed to fly in the face of what we felt was right. We didn't want to be called heroes, but a little consideration would have been nice. We hadn't been goofing off or running away on vacation for seven months either, which was how it seemed some folks treated our absence. And would people please stop asking stupid questions.

"No, I did not kill anyone," said Gunny Grant, "but if I had, do you think I would want to tell you about it at a party? What are these people thinking?"

"It's weird being back," said HM2 Garcia. "I walked into a 7-Eleven the other day, and just grabbed a juice and walked out. I was halfway through the parking lot before I realized what I had done. Luckily, the clerk hadn't noticed. I went back to pay later. I realized I hadn't used money in six months. I had gotten out of the habit."

The barbecue ended, and we all went back to our lives. There were things to do after all: bills to pay, yards to keep up, things to buy, communication problems to improve, projects to manage. All those things that had appeared so trivial in Iraq were piling up into the necessity of everyday life. Even friendships I had forged in Iraq, some of the closest of my life, were taking a back seat to the pressure to keep up. And everything seemed harder now.

The virtual reality project became a source of conflict. We were gathering final results for presentation, and the issue of authorship came up. Perhaps my memory of it was wrong, but I had thought that when I took on running the project it was understood that I would write the "big" paper at the end. Now that plan was challenged. The VR wasn't my idea after all. I hadn't even been around for the past six months. Other than a figurehead, what was my role in the project anyway?

I exploded. I was on this project for three years before I deployed, and no one complained about it then. If I knew it was going to be taken out of my hands at the end, would I really have volunteered to take on ten to twenty hours a week of administrative work, endless political wrangling, and managing two teams that couldn't agree that the sky was blue? I had given up two other perfectly good research projects for this and without getting paid. If I had moonlighted the same number of hours, I would be at least a hundred and fifty thousand dollars richer. I had other issues I needed to deal with: a job, my home, my marriage. Now some podunk statistician, someone who had never seen a patient, who had never set foot on base, and who had gotten paid to work on the project, now he didn't want to turn over a database? Who did these people think they were?

Of course, "who these people were" was the team who had brought the virtual reality idea to us in the first place. They were academics for whom authorship on a publication was far more important than it was to me. The debate over who should control the project, its originator or its manager, was a legitimate one. In calmer times, I probably still would have felt that I was in the right, but its importance would not have been so magnified. I would have remembered that the purpose of the project wasn't to get our names on a scientific publication. It was to help Service Members with PTSD.

War heightens everything. It requires quick reactions and a sense of moral clarity. It's not always easy to come back down from this battlefield mind-set. It's not even always clear that you would want to.

"I went to war with a certain contract in my mind," a patient with PTSD would later tell me, while explaining his struggle to have his condition recognized by the VA. "I didn't expect to be treated as a hero or receive any special favors. But I thought that if I did the right thing by volunteering to go to war, then others would do right by me. So I come back, and there is something wrong with my head. OK, that happens. So why doesn't the Army see it? Why does my wife leave me? I got screwed for doing the right thing, and I want someone to stand up and acknowledge that."

War or no war, civilian life goes on the way it always does. It has its blessings, and its imperfections. No matter what you think you know, or whatever your pain may teach you, the rest of the world cannot see through your eyes. Its view will be what it always was. People will care about their own problems and have their own questions. Academics have their petty squabbles, and courts want you to pay tickets on time. Unfortunately, this means that you have to deal with your own inner demons.

We train to go to war. We spend months or years gaining a particular mind-set, practicing repeatedly the "right" way to react in combat. But there is no training to come home, and no single home to come back to. There are many paths to take. One can take risks or retreat into a safer shell. A person can get angry, be sad, or be grateful for what he or she has at home. In the end, it is true that others should care about helping a Veteran adapt, but sometimes they won't. There is the choice to hold on to that righteous sense of anger or to let it go and try to move on.

I did not accomplish the growth I thought I would when I came home. I did not set aside the material world or devote myself to my friends and family as I thought I should. One of the scientific papers on our virtual reality work went back and forth in authorship, depending mostly on who could get it published. Some of its authors stayed friends. Some of us did not. Mark and Brenda Wiederhold offered me the chance to author a different journal article, one I had not expected to get. They were very generous. Life itself had been generous, and I was finally lucky enough to realize that.

I found a job, replanted my fruit trees, worked on my marriage, and had a son. I didn't set out to finish this book right away. It languished for almost a year. However, you are reading it now. Through luck or providence, I managed to come home unharmed. I was not injured. I do not have post traumatic stress disorder. I was lucky. I was blessed.

I also didn't come back with a magical understanding of how PTSD works or how some Veterans grow as people after their deployments. I did learn that war changes us all, and that we can't always predict how those changes will happen. I learned how important it is that we all come home.

# 18

# A Kind of Peace

## What We Learned and What We Have Left to Accomplish

THE baby is crying when I wake up. I was dreaming of Iraq, and the sound snaps me away from desert sands. Another kind of sand is rubbed out of my eyes, and I pick him up before he wakes my wife. It's not time for his feeding yet. It's just hot. It must be what caused both his awakening and my dreams.

My son was born almost two years to the day after my return date from Iraq. I would have been going back on deployment about now, likely to Afghanistan, if I had stayed in the service. However, I left the Navy within a couple of weeks of returning home. Naval Medical Center San Diego hired me to stay on as a civilian. After that I rejoined the Navy Reserve. A one-weekend-a-month warrior, that's me now. Technically, I could get called back to deploy, but it seems unlikely. Life is pretty peaceful for me. But the war still goes on.

Maddux—that's my son—has been sleeping in our room. We set up a separate space for him, but it has been hard to let go. We're overprotective. I rock him and walk out into the hallway and into what will one day be his bedroom. He calms quickly.

I've decorated the walls of his room with some of the things I loved in childhood, pictures of dragons and comic book heroes. I hope Maddux

likes them. I hope he grows up to believe in heroes and not just those
who wear capes and costumes. I hope he'll understand that Captain
America and Superman exist in real life, even if they are vulnerable to
more than kryptonite.

Comic books taught me a lot as a kid. They taught me to believe in
technology and that good can win in the end. They taught me to believe
that dragons can be tamed and that fierce creatures can be our most important defenders. I also know that these stories can be filled with stuff
and nonsense. There was never any blood when the Lone Ranger shot
someone. Keep an open mind, but not so open that your brain falls out.

We've been trying to be more rigorous in our testing of virtual reality
treatments since I got back from Iraq. Our anecdotal evidence had been
good, but any snake oil salesman on late-night TV can find someone for
whom his product was a "miracle cure." It turned out that my results
in Iraq with VR weren't any better than Dr. Barnum achieved without the simulator. Stateside, however, the virtual reality seemed to have
advantages over traditional treatment. We completed what's called a randomized trial. Twenty patients from Naval Medical Center and Camp
Pendleton came in. They were randomly divided into two groups. Ten
patients received virtual reality treatment. Ten went back to the regular
clinic.

It was a pretty sick group to start out with, so perhaps it wasn't surprising that only one out of the ten who went back to the clinic got
better. Well, one out of nine. One guy didn't come back, so we don't
really know what happened to him. We got luckier with those in virtual
reality. All came back, and seven of them were better. That's what the
scientific world calls "statistically significant," in other words, too big a
difference to be accounted for by random chance. Hurray for us. It got us
on the front page of the American Psychiatric Association's newsletter.
It didn't help the three people who went through the simulator and still
had nightmares. We owe our Service Members more.

I'd like to hope that by the time Maddux is grown there will be no
more war, or sickness, mental or otherwise. That is a pipe dream, but we
are going to keep trying to make things better. We are testing all kinds
of new treatments now, not only virtual reality. A researcher from the
University of San Diego gave us a computer program that is supposed

to help out even if you don't have access to a therapist. We're testing it. We're also testing new medications and new forms of therapy. We're testing simple ideas, such as if you improve sleep does it make therapy more effective overall. We're also testing complex ideas, such as allowing patients to view their own brainwaves during treatment, or altering those brainwaves using very powerful magnets. We are looking at genetics and brain scans and what allows some people to go through the worst of times and come out stronger. We're even making plans to test some pretty "out there" ideas.

An anesthesiologist from Chicago showed us that a shot in the neck that is usually used to treat pain can also dramatically change PTSD symptoms. Right now, it doesn't appear that improvements last, but the treatment enabled one man who had spent two years locked in his home, feeling as though his life wasn't worth living, to get out and enjoy a week with his family. That was encouraging. We are even trying acupuncture and tapping over areas of the body supposedly associated with energy fields. I don't think the last couple of ideas are going anywhere, but there are many people who believe. I'm at least willing to give them a try at scientific inquiry. Like I said, keep an open mind, but not so open that your brain falls out.

We are also investigating more about the virtual reality. A healthy skepticism has to be at the center of scientific medicine. Otherwise, we would all still be using bleeding and leeches. Science demands that facts hold up under repetition, so we are conducting another randomized study of the virtual reality therapy. Other groups are also trying to reproduce the work, with some slight variations. Some are using detailed simulators. Dr. Spira, now at the National Center for PTSD in Honolulu, is looking at the fast versus the slow approach. A group at Madigan Army Medical Center is doing a much-larger randomized study. In San Diego, we're focusing on whether the simulator is really needed or whether we can accomplish the same result with less technology.

This time around we are treating more Service Members. We are putting more therapists to work. This includes veterans of the program such as Dr. Deal, Dr. Johnston, and me, as well as new, fresh faces. Two of our previous research assistants, Alicia Baird and Jennifer Murphy, completed their psychology doctorates and started providing virtual

reality treatment with us. More than thirty providers from military facilities came to train on the machines. Some of them are letting us know
how it is working in their clinics. We are opening up treatment to more
people to see how it works outside the large medical centers.

We've also tried to get rid of the things that might have biased us the
first time around. We've divorced ourselves from companies that sell
virtual reality machines. It makes getting technical assistance difficult
if a VR machine breaks down, but we hope it will enable a less biased
result. We've also ensured that people who rate whether patients get
better don't know which treatment the patient received. This is called
*study blinding.* We have made sure that both treatment options include
computers in the treatment, so that the halo of technology isn't what
makes the difference. Most important, we compare virtual reality treatment not only to any old therapy but also to the gold standard for PTSD
treatment. We are sure that our virtual reality mousetrap works, but
now we need to know whether it is a *better* mousetrap.

Even if virtual reality is the best, proven treatment out there, that
would only mean it was true on average. An anatomy teacher once
pointed out to me that the average patient has one testicle and one ovary.
People are not made like math problems. We still need to figure out the
special component that will allow this individual person to thrive.

Maddux falls back asleep as we walk around the comic book characters and dragons of his room. I smile at his smile. I'm reminded of one of
my favorite comic book stories: The protagonist is not a costumed hero
but a character named Morpheus, the living embodiment of dream. In
the comic book, Morpheus does battle with a demon. Both Morpheus
and the demon can transform into anything they imagine: so it is a para-
dox, the unstoppable force versus the immovable object.

They take turns saying what they will change themselves into to de-
feat the other. Morpheus becomes a cat, so the demon becomes a dog.
Morpheus becomes a lion, the demon a hunter, and so on.

Finally, Morpheus, having had enough of this game, decides that he
will become all things, the whole universe.

At this, the demon smiles, thinking he has won. With sharp teeth he
says, "I am Anti-Life, the Beast of Judgment. I am the dark at the end of

everything. The end of universes, gods, worlds . . . of everything. And what will you be *then*, Dreamlord?"

To which the king of dreams, who speaks through older and wiser teeth, replies, "I am hope."

So it was that the demon was defeated.

At least, that is the way it goes in comic books. In real life, defeating the demons of war takes hope and hard work. It takes perseverance, the love and support of friends, the loyalty of comrades in arms. It requires science and technology and medicine. It takes church and synagogue and mosque, a backyard barbeque, and a baseball game. It takes months, sometimes years of therapy. Different things are needed for different people, and all of us require the basics. Sometimes, even hard-nosed skepticism is needed, the type that doubts that a video game could really cure PTSD.

Yet lessons of a children's story are not wrong. I don't know that virtual reality was actually what let people get back to their lives and families after suffering from PTSD. I do know that people who were treated this way got better. I know that hope can win. I know the demons can be defeated and that we can keep our children safe.

Sweet dreams, little Maddux. Sweet dreams to us all.

# Acknowledgments

THANK you to my mother, Barbara McLay, who edited this book and sent it out to publishers when I had given up on it. Everyone should be so lucky as to have someone who believes in you that way. Also, many thanks to the doctors, scientists, teachers, counselors, mentors, Service Members, family, friends, and patients who taught me the lessons presented in this book. Most important, my most profound gratitude to the men and women of America's Armed Forces, who allowed me the honor to serve with them, who brought me home from war alive, and who make every sacrifice to keep us safe and free.

# Index